The Complete Alkaline Diet Cookbook

4 Books in 1| Dr. Lewis's Meal Plan Project| Ultimate Guide on How to Balance Body Acids by Following a Practical, Tasty and Effective Method| 400 Affordable Recipes Without Giving Up Your Favorite Foods

By Grace Lewis

The content contained within this book may not be reproduced, duplicated or transmitted without direct written permission from the author or the publisher.

Under no circumstances will any blame or legal responsibility be held against the publisher, or author, for any damages, reparation, or monetary loss due to the information contained within this book. Either directly or indirectly.

Legal Notice:

This book is copyright protected. This book is only for personal use. You cannot amend, distribute, sell, use, quote or paraphrase any part, or the content within this book, without the consent of the author or publisher.

Disclaimer Notice:

Please note the information contained within this document is for educational and entertainment purpose sonly. All effort has been executed to present accurate, up to date, and reliable, complete information. No warranties of any kind are declared or implied. Readers acknowledge that the author is not engaging in the rendering of legal, financial, medical or professional advice. The content within this book has been derived from various sources. Please consult a licensed professional before attempting any techniques outlined in this book. By reading this document, the reader agrees that under no circumstances is the author responsible for any losses, direct or indirect, which are incurred as a result of the use of information contained within this document, including, but not limited to, - errors, omissions, or inaccuracies.

Copyright © 2021 Grace Lewis

All rights reserved.

ISBN: 978-1-80300-453-2 (Paperback)

ISBN: 978-1-80300-454-9 (Hardcover)

Table of Contents

Alkaline Diet Cookbook for Women

Chapter 1 - Introduction 14

Chapter 2 - Breakfast Recipes 16

   1) Bowl of raspberry and banana smoothie 17
   2) Apple and walnut porridge 17
   3) Chia seed pudding 17
   4) Cauliflower and raspberry porridge 17
   5) Spicy quinoa porridge 17
   6) Chocolate quinoa porridge 18
   7) Buckwheat porridge with walnuts 18
   8) Fruity Oatmeal 19
   9) Baked Walnut Oatmeal 19
   10) Banana Waffles 19
   11) Savory sweet potato waffles 20
   12) Fruit Oatmeal Pancakes 20
   13) Tofu and mushroom muffins 20
   14) Simple white bread 21
   15) Quinoa bread 21
   16) Zucchini and banana bread 21
   17) Granola with coconut, nuts and seeds 22
   18) Tortilla Chips 22
   19) Onion Rings 23
   20) Strawberry Sorbet 23

Chapter 3 - Lunch Recipes 24

   21) Tomato and vegetable salad 25
   22) Cauliflower Soup 25
   23) Tomato Soup 26
   24) Garlic broccoli 26
   25) Curried okra 26
   26) Mushrooms curry 27
   27) Glazed Brussels sprouts 27
   28) Sauteed mushrooms 27
   29) Sweet and sour cabbage 28
   30) Brussels sprouts with walnuts 28
   31) Roasted Butternut Squash 28
   32) Broccoli with peppers 28
   33) Shrimp with tamari 28
   34) Vegetarian Kebab 29
   35) Fried onion sprout 29
   36) Southwestern stuffed sweet potatoes 30
   37) Zoodles with cream sauce 30
   38) Rainbow Pad Thai 30
   39) Lentils and vegetables 30
   40) Vegetable dish with sesame 31

Chapter 4 - Dinner Recipes 32

   41) Stew without beef 33
   42) Emmenthal soup 33
   43) Spaghetti with broccoli 33
   44) Indian Lentil Curry 34
   45) Vegetables with wild rice 34
   46) Spicy Lentil Soup 34
   47) Leek soup with mushrooms 35
   48) Fresh vegetarian pizza 35
   49) Spicy Lentil Burger 35
   50) Roasted cauliflower rolls 36
   51) Sliced sweet potato with artichoke cream and peppers 36
   52) Cooking scallops, onions and potatoes 37

53)	Spicy cilantro and coconut soup	37		78)	Hummus	45
54)	Tarragon soup	37		79)	Paleo vegan zucchini hummus	46
55)	Asparagus and artichoke soup	38		80)	German style sweet potato salad	46
56)	Mint and berry soup	38		Chapter 6 -	Dessert Recipes	48
57)	Mushroom soup	38		81)	Red fruit and vegetable smoothie	48
58)	Potato and lentil stew	39		82)	Kale Smoothie	48
59)	Mixed mushroom stew	39		83)	Green Tofu Smoothie	48
60)	Mixed stew of spicy vegetables	39		84)	Grape and chard smoothie	48
Chapter 5 -	Snacks Recipes	40		85)	Matcha Smoothie	49
61)	Bean burgers	41		86)	Banana Smoothie	49
62)	Grilled watermelon	41		87)	Strawberry Smoothie	49
63)	Mango sauce	41		88)	Raspberry and tofu smoothie	49
64)	Avocado gazpacho	41		89)	Mango Smoothie	50
65)	Roasted chickpeas	41		90)	Pineapple Smoothie	50
66)	Banana chips	42		91)	Cabbage and pineapple smoothie	50
67)	Roasted cashews	42		92)	Green Vegetable Smoothie	50
68)	Dried orange slices	42		93)	Avocado and spinach smoothie	51
69)	Chickpea hummus	43		94)	Cucumber Smoothie	51
70)	Avocado chips in the oven	43		95)	Apple and Ginger Smoothie	51
71)	Dried apples with cinnamon	43		96)	Green Tea Blueberry Smoothie	51
72)	Guacamole sauce	43		97)	Apple and almond smoothie	52
73)	Apple chip	44		98)	Cranberry Smoothie	52
74)	Alka-Goulash fast	44		99)	Berry and Cinnamon Smoothie	52
75)	Eggplant Caviar	44		100)	Detoxifying Berry Smoothie	52
76)	Spiced nut mixture	45		Chapter 7 -	Dr. Lewis's Meal Plan Project	53
77)	Garlic mushrooms	45		Chapter 8 -	Conclusion	54

Alkaline Diet Cookbook for Men

Chapter 1 - Introduction 56

Chapter 2 - Breakfast Recipes 58

1) Blueberry Muffins 59
2) Banana Strawberry Ice Crem 59
3) Chocolate cream Homemade Whipped 60
4) "Chocolate" Pudding 60
5) Walnut muffins 60
6) Banana and almond smoothie 61
7) Strawberry and Beet Smoothie 61
8) Raspberry and tofu smoothie 61
9) Mango and lemon smoothie 61
10) Papaya and banana smoothie 62
11) Orange and Oat Smoothie 62
12) Pineapple and Kale Smoothie 62
13) Pumpkin and Banana Smoothie 62
14) Cabbage and avocado smoothie 63
15) Cucumber and Herb Smoothie 63
16) Hemp seed and carrot muffins 63
17) Chia seed and strawberry parfait 64
18) Pecan Pancakes 64
19) Quinoa Breakfast 64
20) Oatmeal 65

Chapter 3 - Lunch Recipes 66

21) Sweet spinach salad 67
22) Steamed green bowl 67
23) Vegetable and berry salad 67
24) Bowl of quinoa and carrots 68
25) Grab and Go Wraps 68
26) Walnut Tacos 68
27) Tex-Mex bowl 69

28) Avocado and salmon soup 69
29) Asian Pumpkin Salad 70
30) Sweet potato rolls 70
31) Spicy cabbage bowl 70
32) Citrus and fennel salad 71
33) Vegan Burger 71
34) Alkaline spicy cabbage 71
35) Electric Salad 72
36) Kale salad 72
37) Walnut, date, orange and cabbage salad .. 72
38) Tomatoes with basil-snack 73
39) Pasta with spelt, zucchini and eggplant 73
40) Alkalizing millet dish 73

Chapter 4 - Dinner Recipes 74

41) Mixed stew of spicy vegetables 75
42) Mixed vegetable stew with herbs 75
43) Tofu and bell pepper stew 75
44) Roasted Pumpkin Curry 75
45) Lentils, vegetables and apple curry 76
46) Curried red beans 76
47) Lentil and Carrot Chili 76
48) Black beans with chilli 77
49) Cook mixed vegetables 77
50) Vegetarian Ratatouille 77
51) Quinoa with vegetables 78
52) Lentils with cabbage 78
53) Lentils with tomatoes 79
54) Spicy baked beans 79
55) Chickpeas with pumpkin 79
56) Chickpeas with cabbage 79

57)	Stuffed cabbage rolls	80
58)	Green beans and mushrooms in casserole	81
59)	Meatloaf of wild rice and lentils	81
60)	Vegetable soup and spelt noodles	82

Chapter 5 - Snacks Recipes 84

61)	Quinoa Salad	84
62)	Almonds with sautéed vegetables	84
63)	Alkaline Sweet Potato Mash	84
64)	Mediterranean peppers	84
65)	Tomato and avocado sauce with potatoes	85
66)	Alkaline beans and coconut	85
67)	Alkalized vegetable lasagna	85
68)	Aloo Gobi	86
69)	Chocolate Crunch Bars	86
70)	Nut Butter Bars	86
71)	Homemade Protein Bar	86
72)	Shortbread Coookies	86
73)	Coconut cookies Chip	87
74)	Coconut Cookies	87
75)	Berry Mousse	87
76)	Coconut pulp Coookies	87
77)	Avocado Pudding	88
78)	Coconut Raisins cooookies	88
79)	Cracker Pumpkin Spice	88
80)	Spicy Toasted nuts	88

Chapter 6 - Dessert Recipes 90

81)	Cracker Healthy	91
82)	Tortillas	91
83)	Walnut cheesecake Mango	91
84)	Blackberry Jam	92
85)	Blackberry Bars	92
86)	Squash Pie.	92
87)	Walnut Milk homemade	93
88)	Aquafaba	93
89)	Milk Homemade Hempsed	94
90)	Oil spicy infusion	94
91)	Italian infused oil	94
92)	Garlic Infused Oil	94
93)	Papaya Seeds Mango Dressing	95
94)	Blueberry Smoothie	95
95)	Raspberry and tofu smoothie	95
96)	Beet and Strawberry Smoothie	95
97)	Kiwi Smoothie	96
98)	Pineapple and Carrot Smoothie	96
99)	Oatmeal and orange smoothie	96
100)	Pumpkin Smoothie	96

Chapter 7 - Dr. Lewis's Meal Plan Project 97

Chapter 8 - Conclusion 98

Alkaline Diet Cookbook for Athletes

Chapter 1 - Introduction 100

Chapter 2 - Breakfast Recipes 102

1) Baked Grapefruit 103
2) Almond Fritters 103
3) Amaranth Porridge 103
4) Banana Porridge 103
5) Zucchini Muffins 104
6) Tofu Stew With Vegetables 104
7) Zucchini Fritters 104
8) Pumpkin Quinoa 104
9) Avocado Toast 105
10) Frozen Banana Breakfast Bowl 105
11) Cobbler Of Chia Seeds And Blueberries 105
12) Quick And Easy Granola Bars 106
13) Alkaline Blueberry Spelt Pancakes 106
14) Blueberry Alkaline Muffins 106
15) Meal Of Crispy Quinoa 107
16) Coconut Pancakes 107
17) Quinoa Porridge 107
18) Amaranth Porridge 107
19) Banana Barley Porridge 108
20) Zucchini Muffins 108

Chapter 3 - Lunch Recipes 110

21) Green Noodle Salad 111
22) Pumpkin Ratatouille 111
23) Roasted Vegetables 111
24) Crockpot Summer Vegetables 112
25) Brazilian Cabbage 112
26) Algae Wraps With Quinoa And Vegetables 112
27) Lettuce Wraps 113
28) Rainbow Salad With Meyer Lemon Dressing . 113
29) Alkaline Quinoa & Hummus Wraps 113
30) Grilled Zucchini Salad 114
31) Creamy Cabbage Salad With Avocado And Tomato 114
32) Rice With Sesame And Ginger 114
33) Macaroni And 'Cheese 115
34) Creamy Kamut Pasta 115
35) Basil Avocado Pasta 116
36) Jamaican Jerk Patties 116
37) Kamut Patties 117
38) Mushroom Burgers Portobello 117
39) Healthy Fried-Rice 117
40) Veg-Meatballs 118

Chapter 4 - Dinner Recipes 120

41) Cabbage, Soursop And Zucchini Soup 121
42) Green Chickpea Soup 121
43) Green Zucchini Soup 121
44) Kamut Vegetable Soup With Tarragon 122
45) Pumpkin Soup With Basil 122
46) Coconut Mushroom Soup 122
47) Onion And Pumpkin Soup 123
48) Chayote Mushroom And Hemp Milk Stew 123
49) Coconut Soup With Butternut Squash 123
50) Mushroom And Tomato Coconut Soup 124
51) Curried Cabbage And Chickpeas 124
52) Coconut And Cashew Soup With Tarragon ... 124
53) Cucumber And Zucchini Soup 125
54) Coconut Soup With Jalapeno And Lime 125
55) Watermelon And Jalapeno Gazpacho 125
56) Carrot And Fennel Soup 125

57) Coconut Stew With Lentils And Herb Potatoes 126

58) Cauliflower And Roasted Garlic Soup............ 126

59) Carrot And Potato Stew With Herbs 126

60) Berry And Mint Soup................................. 127

Chapter 5 - Snacks Recipes 128

61) Wheat Crackers 129

62) Chips Potato 129

63) Zucchini Pepper Chips............................. 129

64) Flat Bread 129

65) Cracker Healthy 130

66) Tortillas... 130

67) Walnut Cheesecake Mango 130

68) Blackberry Jam 131

69) Blackberry Bars..................................... 131

70) SqUash Pie. 131

71) Walnut Milk Homemade 132

72) AqUafaba.. 132

73) Milk Homemade Hempsed 132

74) Oil Spicy Infusion 132

75) Italian Infused Oil.................................. 133

76) Garlic Infused Oil 133

77) Papaya Seeds Mango Dressing................. 133

78) Blueberry Smoothie 133

79) Raspberry And Tofu Smoothie 134

80) Beet And Strawberry Smoothie 134

Chapter 6 - Dessert Recipes 136

81) Kiwi Smoothie 137

82) Pineapple And Carrot Smoothie 137

83) Oatmeal And Orange Smoothie................. 137

84) Pumpkin Smoothie 137

85) Red Fruit And Vegetable Smoothie............ 138

86) Kale Smoothie 138

87) Green Tofu Smoothie 138

88) Grape And Chard Smoothie 138

89) Matcha Smoothie................................... 139

90) Banana Smoothie 139

91) Strawberry Smoothie 139

92) Raspberry And Tofu Smoothie 139

93) Mango Smoothie................................... 140

94) Pineapple Smoothie 140

95) Cabbage And Pineapple Smoothie............. 140

96) Green Vegetable Smoothie 140

97) Avocado And Spinach Smoothie................ 141

98) Cucumber Smoothie............................... 141

99) Apple And Ginger Smoothie 141

100) Green Tea Blueberry Smoothie................ 141

Chapter 7 - Dr. Lewis's Meal Plan Project.............. 142

Chapter 8 - Conclusion 143

Alkaline Diet Cookbook on a Budget

Chapter 1 - Introduction 145

Chapter 2 - Breakfast Recipes 146

1) Mile Porridge 147
2) Jackfruit Fry vegetable 147
3) Zucchini Pancakes 147
4) Squash Hash 147
5) Hemp Seed Porridge 148
6) Veggie Medley 148
7) Pumpkin Spice Quinoa 148
8) Coconut pulp Coookies 148
9) Avocado Pudding 149
10) Coconut Raisins cooookies 149
11) Cracker Pumpkin Spice 149
12) Spicy Toasted nuts 149
13) Wheat Crackers 150
14) Chips potato 150
15) Zucchini Pepper Chips 150
16) Flat bread 150
17) Cracker Healthy 151
18) Tortillas 151
19) Pink Smoothie 151
20) Green Apple Smoothie 151

Chapter 3 - Lunch Recipes 152

21) Roasted artichoke salad 153
22) Artichoke pie 153
23) Vegetable fritters 153
24) Mint and lime salad 154
25) Zucchini salad 154
26) Fried tofu 154
27) Potato and pumpkin meatballs 155
28) Italian soffritto 155
29) Southern Salad 155
30) Roasted vegetables 156
31) Pad Thai Salad 156
32) Cucumber salad 156
33) Pasta salad with red lentils 157
34) Salad with peach sauce 157
35) Pineapple salad 157
36) Sweet potato salad with Jalapeno sauce 158
37) Asparagus salad with lemon sauce 158
38) Vegetarian lettuce rolls 159
39) Oatmeal, tofu and spinach burger 159
40) Hamburger with beans, nuts and vegetables. 159

Chapter 4 - Dinner Recipes 160

41) Potato and broccoli soup 161
42) Lush bell pepper soup 161
43) Cabbage and yellow onion soup 161
44) Wild rice, mushroom and leek soup 162
45) Pear and ginger soup 162
46) Asparagus and artichoke soup 162
47) Carrot and celery soup 163
48) Creamy clam chowder with mushrooms 163
49) Soup of bok choy, broccolini and brown rice. 163
50) Apple and sweet pumpkin soup 164
51) Tomato and carrot soup with lemon 164
52) Zucchini and avocado soup with basil 164
53) Zucchini, spinach and quinoa soup 165
54) Easy Cilantro Lime Quinoa 165
55) Spinach Quinoa 165
56) Healthy broccoli soup Asparagus 166

57)	Creamy Asparagus Soup	166
58)	Spicy Eggplant	166
59)	Brussels Sprouts and carrots	167
60)	Cajun Zucchini seasoned	167

Chapter 5 -   Snacks Recipes 168

61)	Cracker Healthy	169
62)	Tortillas	169
63)	Walnut cheesecake Mango	169
64)	Blackberry Jam	169
65)	Blackberry Bars	170
66)	Squash Pie	170
67)	Walnut Milk homemade	170
68)	Aquafaba	171
69)	Milk Homemade Hempsed	171
70)	Oil spicy infusion	171
71)	Italian infused oil	171
72)	Garlic Infused Oil	172
73)	Papaya Seeds Mango Dressing	172
74)	Blueberry Smoothie	172
75)	Raspberry and tofu smoothie	172
76)	Beet and Strawberry Smoothie	173
77)	Kiwi Smoothie	173
78)	Pineapple and Carrot Smoothie	173
79)	Oatmeal and orange smoothie	173
80)	Pumpkin Smoothie	174

Chapter 6 -   Dessert Recipes 176

81)	Red fruit and vegetable smoothie	177
82)	Kale Smoothie	177
83)	Green Tofu Smoothie	177
84)	Grape and chard smoothie	177
85)	Matcha Smoothie	178
86)	Banana Smoothie	178
87)	Strawberry Smoothie	178
88)	Raspberry and tofu smoothie	178
89)	Mango Smoothie	179
90)	Pineapple Smoothie	179
91)	Cabbage and pineapple smoothie	179
92)	Green Vegetable Smoothie	179
93)	Avocado and spinach smoothie	180
94)	Cucumber Smoothie	180
95)	Apple and Ginger Smoothie	180
96)	Green Tea Blueberry Smoothie	180
97)	Apple and almond smoothie	181
98)	Cranberry Smoothie	181
99)	Berry and Cinnamon Smoothie	181
100)	Detoxifying Berry Smoothie	181

Chapter 7 -   Chapter 7 - Dr. Lewis's Meal Plan Project 182

Chapter 8 -   Chapter 8 - Conclusion 183

Alkaline Diet Cookbook for Women

Dr. Lewis's Meal Plan Project | How to Make Your Body Ready for Weight Loss by Balancing Acidic and Alkaline Foods

By Grace Lewis

Chapter 1 - Introduction

The alkaline diet is based on the consideration that a diet rich in acid foods ends up disturbing the acid-base balance of the body, promoting the loss of essential minerals, such as calcium and magnesium contained in the bones.

These alterations would favor the appearance of a chronic acidosis of mild degree, which in turn would be a predisposing factor for some diseases and for a general sense of malaise.

The alkaline diet recommends to consume 70-80% of alkaline foods and 20-30% of acid foods every day. This food model is much closer to the one followed by man until the discovery of agriculture than the current one.

The acidity of a food is not measured in its fresh state, but on the ashes (minerals) that remain after combustion. These inorganic substances, therefore not metabolizable, can behave as acids or bases, and as such participate in the maintenance of the normal organic pH.

Lemon, for example, has a very low pH, because of the abundant presence of citric acid; however, it is considered as an alkaline food because its acid components have an organic nature and as such they are easily metabolized by the body and eliminated with respiration, whereas the basic inorganic ones remain there for a longer time.

The elements that cause the formation of acids, by decreasing the urinary pH, are sulfur, phosphor and chlorine, whereas foods rich in sodium, potassium, magnesium and calcium are considered alkaline.

What do you eat on an alkaline diet?

The alkaline diet basically reinforces good, old-fashioned healthy eating. The diet recommends eating more vegetables, fruits and drinking plenty of water and cutting back on sugar, alcohol, meat and processed foods.

Where to start with the alkaline diet?

In this book you will find targeted recipes and especially easy to prepare to be able to approach the alkaline diet at its best.

At the end of the book you'll find my personal meal plan developed specifically for women, so that you can immediately experience the fantastic benefits that this diet can bring you.

Good luck and... Bon appetite!

Grace

Chapter 2 - Breakfast Recipes

1) Bowl of raspberry and banana smoothie

Preparation time: 10 minutes   **Cooking time:** 10 minutes   **Servings:** 2

Ingredients:
- 2 cups fresh raspberries, split
- 2 large frozen bananas, peeled

Ingredients:
- ½ cup of unsweetened almond milk
- 1/3 cup fresh mixed berries

Directions:
- In a blender, add the raspberries, bananas and almond milk and blend until smooth.
- Transfer the smoothie to two serving bowls evenly.
- Top each bowl with berries and serve immediately.

Nutrition: Calories

2) Apple and walnut porridge

Preparation time: 10 minutes   **Cooking time:** 5 minutes   **Servings:** 4

Ingredients:
- 2 cups of unsweetened almond milk
- 3 tablespoons walnuts, chopped
- 3 tablespoons of sunflower seeds
- 2 large apples, peeled, pitted and grated

Ingredients:
- ½ teaspoon of organic vanilla extract
- Pinch of cinnamon powder
- ½ small apple, core and slices
- 1 small banana, peeled and sliced

Directions:
- In a large skillet, stir together the milk, nuts, sunflower seeds, applesauce, vanilla and cinnamon over medium-low heat and cook for about 3-5 minutes, stirring often.
- Remove from heat and transfer oatmeal to serving bowls.
- Top with apple and banana slices and serve.

Nutrition: Calories

3) Chia seed pudding

Preparation time: 10 minutes   **Cooking time:** 10 minutes   **Servings:** 3

Ingredients:
- 2 cups of unsweetened almond milk
- ½ cup chia seeds
- 1 tablespoon maple syrup

Ingredients:
- 1 teaspoon of organic vanilla extract
- 1/3 cup fresh strawberries, hulled and sliced
- 2 tablespoons of sliced almonds

Directions:
- In a large bowl, add the almond milk, chia seeds, maple syrup and vanilla extract and stir to combine well.
- Cover the bowl and refrigerate for at least 3-4 hours, stirring occasionally.
- Serve with the strawberry and almond garnish.

Nutrition: Calories

4) Cauliflower and raspberry porridge

Preparation time: 10 minutes   **Cooking time:** 15 minutes   **Servings:** 2

Ingredients:
- 1 cup unsweetened coconut milk
- 1 cup cauliflower rice
- 1/3 cup fresh raspberries

Ingredients:
- 3 tablespoons unsweetened coconut, shredded
- 3 drops of liquid stevia

Directions:
- In a skillet, add the coconut milk and cauliflower rice over medium heat and cook for about 2-3 minutes, stirring occasionally.
- Add the raspberries and with the back of a spoon lightly crush them.
- Add the coconut and stevia and stir to combine.
- Cover the pan and cook for about 10 minutes, stirring occasionally.
- Serve hot.

Nutrition: Calories

5) Spicy quinoa porridge

Preparation time: 10 minutes   **Cooking time:** 15 minutes   **Servings:** 4

Ingredients:
- ✓ 1 cup uncooked, rinsed and drained red quinoa
- ✓ 2 cups of alkaline water
- ✓ ½ teaspoon of organic vanilla extract
- ✓ ½ cup of coconut milk

Directions:
- ❖ In a large skillet, mix the quinoa, water and vanilla extract over medium heat and bring to a boil.
- ❖ Reduce heat to low and simmer, covered for about 15 minutes or until all liquid is absorbed, stirring occasionally.

Nutrition: Calories

Ingredients:
- ✓ ¼ teaspoon fresh lemon peel, finely grated
- ✓ 10-12 drops of liquid stevia
- ✓ 1 teaspoon of cinnamon powder
- ✓ ½ teaspoon ground ginger
- ✓ Pinch of ground cloves
- ✓ 2 tablespoons of chopped almonds
- ❖ In the pan with the quinoa, add the coconut milk, lemon zest, stevia and spices and stir to combine.
- ❖ Immediately remove from heat and stir quinoa with a fork.
- ❖ Divide the quinoa mixture evenly among the serving bowls.
- ❖ Serve with a garnish of chopped almonds.

6) *Chocolate quinoa porridge*

Preparation time: 15 minutes   **Cooking time:** 30 minutes   **Servings:** 4

Ingredients:
- ✓ 1 cup uncooked quinoa, rinsed and drained
- ✓ 1 cup unsweetened almond milk
- ✓ 1 cup unsweetened coconut milk
- ✓ Pinch of sea salt

Directions:
- ❖ Heat a small nonstick skillet over medium heat and cook quinoa for about 3 minutes or until lightly toasted, stirring often.
- ❖ Add the almond milk, coconut milk and a pinch of salt and stir to combine.
- ❖ Increase heat to high and bring to a boil.

Nutrition: Calories

Ingredients:
- ✓ 2 spoons of cocoa powder
- ✓ 2 tablespoons of maple syrup
- ✓ ½ teaspoon of organic vanilla extract
- ✓ ½ cup fresh strawberries, hulled and sliced
- ❖ Reduce heat to low and cook, uncovered for about 20-25 minutes or until all liquid is absorbed, stirring occasionally.
- ❖ Remove from heat and immediately, stir in the cocoa powder, maple syrup and vanilla extract.
- ❖ Serve immediately with the garnish of strawberry slices.

7) *Buckwheat porridge with walnuts*

Preparation time: 15 minutes   **Cooking time:** 7 minutes   **Servings:** 2

Ingredients:
- ✓ ½ cup buckwheat
- ✓ 1 cup of alkaline water
- ✓ 2 tablespoons of chia seeds
- ✓ 15-20 almonds
- ✓ 1 cup unsweetened almond milk

Directions:
- ❖ In a large bowl, soak buckwheat groats in water overnight.
- ❖ In 2 other bowls, dip chia seeds and almonds, respectively.
- ❖ Drain the buckwheat and rinse well.
- ❖ In a nonstick skillet, add buckwheat and almond milk over medium heat and cook for about 7 minutes or until creamy.

Nutrition: Calories

Ingredients:
- ✓ ½ teaspoon of cinnamon powder
- ✓ 1 teaspoon of organic vanilla extract
- ✓ 3-4 drops of liquid stevia
- ✓ ¼ cup fresh mixed berries

- ❖ Drain chia seeds and almonds well.
- ❖ Remove the pan from the heat and stir in the almonds, chia seeds, cinnamon, vanilla extract and stevia.
- ❖ Serve warm with a berry garnish.

8) Fruity Oatmeal

Preparation time: 15 minutes   **Cooking time**: 10 minutes   **Servings**: 4

Ingredients:
- 4 cups of alkaline water
- 1 cup steel cut dry oats
- 1 large banana, peeled and mashed

Ingredients:
- 1½ cups of fresh mixed berries (your choice)
- ¼ cup walnuts, finely chopped

Directions:
- In a large skillet, add the water and oats over medium-high heat and bring to a boil.
- Reduce the heat to low and simmer for about 20 minutes, stirring occasionally.
- Remove from heat and cool slightly.
- Add the mashed banana and stir to combine.
- Top with strawberries and walnuts and serve.

Nutrition: Calories

9) Baked Walnut Oatmeal

Preparation time: 15 minutes   **Cooking time**: 45 minutes   **Servings**: 5

Ingredients:
- 1 tablespoon of flaxseed meal
- 3 tablespoons of alkaline water
- 3 cups of unsweetened almond milk
- ¼ cup maple syrup
- 2 tablespoons of coconut oil, melted and cooled
- 2 teaspoons of organic vanilla extract

Ingredients:
- 1 teaspoon of cinnamon powder
- 1 teaspoon of organic baking powder
- ¼ teaspoon of sea salt
- 2 cups of old rolled oats
- ½ cup almonds, chopped
- ½ cup walnuts, chopped

Directions:
- Lightly grease an 8x8-inch baking dish. Set aside.
- In a large bowl, add the flaxseed meal and water and beat until well combined. Set aside for about 5 minutes.
- In the bowl of the flax mixture, add the remaining ingredients except the oats and nuts and mix until well combined.
- Add the oats and nuts and stir gently to combine.
- Place the mixture in the prepared baking dish and spread it out in an even layer.
- Cover the pan with plastic wrap and refrigerate for about 8 hours.
- Preheat the oven to 350 degrees F. Arrange a rack in the center of the oven.
- Remove the pan from the refrigerator and let rest at room temperature for 15-20 minutes.
- Remove the plastic wrap and mix the oatmeal mixture well.
- Bake for about 45 minutes.
- Remove from oven and set aside to cool slightly.
- Serve hot.

Nutrition: Calories

10) Banana Waffles

Preparation time: 15 minutes   **Cooking time**: 20 minutes   **Servings**: 5

Ingredients:
- 2 tablespoons of flax meal
- 6 tablespoons of warm alkaline water
- 2 bananas, peeled and mashed

Ingredients:
- 1 cup creamy almond butter
- ¼ cup whole coconut milk

Directions:
- In a small bowl, add the flax meal and warm water and whisk until well combined.
- Set aside for about 10 minutes or until mixture becomes thick.
- In a medium bowl, add bananas, almond butter and coconut milk, mix well.
- Add the flax meal mixture and stir until well combined.
- Preheat the waffle iron and grease it lightly.
- Place desired amount of batter in preheated waffle iron.
- Bake for about 3-4 minutes or until waffles turn golden brown.
- Repeat with the remaining mixture.
- Serve hot.

Nutrition: Calories

11) Savory sweet potato waffles

Preparation time: 10 minutes Cooking time: 20 minutes Servings: 2

Ingredients:
- 1 medium sweet potato, peeled, grated and squeezed
- 1 teaspoon fresh thyme, chopped
- 1 teaspoon fresh rosemary, chopped

Ingredients:
- 1/8 teaspoon of red pepper flakes, crushed
- Sea salt and freshly ground black pepper, to taste

Directions:
- Preheat the waffle iron and then grease it.
- In a large bowl, add all ingredients and mix until well combined.
- Place ½ of the sweet potato mixture into the preheated waffle iron and bake for about 8-10 minutes or until golden brown.
- Repeat with the remaining mixture.
- Serve hot.

Nutrition: Calories

12) Fruit Oatmeal Pancakes

Preparation time: 10 minutes Cooking time: 15 minutes Servings: 3

Ingredients:
- 1 cup rolled oats
- 1 medium banana, peeled and mashed
- ¼-½ cup unsweetened almond milk
- 1 tablespoon of organic baking powder

Ingredients:
- 1 tablespoon organic apple cider vinegar
- 1 tablespoon of agave nectar
- ½ teaspoon of organic vanilla extract
- ½ cup of fresh blackberries

Directions:
- Place all ingredients except blackberries in a large bowl and mix until well combined.
- Gently add the blackberries.
- Set the mixture aside for about 5-10 minutes.
- Preheat a large nonstick skillet over medium-low heat.
- Add about ¼ cup of the mixture and using a spatula, spread into an even layer.
- Immediately, cover the pan and cook for about 2-3 minutes or until golden brown.
- Flip the pancake and bake for another 1-2 minutes or until golden brown.
- Repeat with the remaining mixture.
- Serve hot.

Nutrition: Calories

13) Tofu and mushroom muffins

Preparation time: 15 minutes Cooking time: 30 minutes Servings: 6

Ingredients:
- 1 teaspoon of olive oil
- 1½ cups fresh button mushrooms, chopped
- 1 shallot, chopped
- 1 teaspoon of minced garlic
- 1 teaspoon fresh rosemary, chopped
- Freshly ground black pepper, to taste

Ingredients:
- 1 (12.3ounce) package of firm silken tofu, drained, pressed and sliced
- ¼ cup unsweetened almond milk
- 2 tablespoons of nutritional yeast
- 1 tablespoon arrowroot starch
- ¼ teaspoon ground turmeric
- 1 teaspoon of coconut oil, softened

Directions:
- Preheat oven to 375 degrees F. Grease a 12-cup muffin pan.
- In a nonstick skillet, heat the oil over medium heat and sauté the shallots and garlic for about 1 minute.
- Add the mushrooms and cook for about 5-7 minutes, stirring often.
- Add the rosemary and black pepper and remove from heat.
- Set aside to cool slightly.
- In a food processor, add the tofu and remaining ingredients and pulse until smooth.
- Transfer the tofu mixture to a large bowl.
- Add the mushroom mixture.
- Divide the tofu mixture evenly among the prepared muffin cups.
- Bake for 20-22 minutes or until a toothpick inserted into the center comes out clean.
- Remove the muffin pan from the oven and place on a rack to cool for about 10 minutes.
- Carefully invert the muffins onto the wire rack and serve warm.

Nutrition: Calories

14) Simple white bread

Preparation time: 10 minutes **Cooking time:** 1 hour and 10 minutes **Servings:** 8

Ingredients:
- 4 cups of spelt flour
- 4 tablespoons of sesame seeds
- 1 teaspoon of baking soda

Ingredients:
- ¼ teaspoon of sea salt
- 10-12 drops of liquid stevia
- 2 cups plus 2 tablespoons of unsweetened almond milk

Directions:
- Preheat oven to 350 degrees F. Line a 9x5-inch baking dish with greased baking paper.
- In a large bowl, add all ingredients and, using a fork, mix until well combined.
- Transfer the mixture to the prepared baking dish evenly.
- Bake for about 70 minutes or until a toothpick inserted into the center comes out clean.
- Remove from the oven and place the pan on a wire rack to cool for at least 10 minutes.
- Carefully flip the loaf onto the rack to cool completely before slicing.
- Using a sharp knife, cut the loaf into desired size slices and serve.

Nutrition: Calories

15) Quinoa bread

Preparation time: 10 minutes **Cooking time:** 1 hour and a half **Servings:** 12

Ingredients:
- ¼ cup chia seeds
- 1 cup of alkaline water, divided by
- 1¾ cups uncooked quinoa, soaked overnight and rinsed
- ½ teaspoon of baking soda

Ingredients:
- ¼ teaspoon of sea salt
- ¼ cup olive oil
- 1 tablespoon fresh lemon juice

Directions:
- In a bowl, soak chia seeds in ½ cup of water overnight,
- Preheat oven to 320 degrees F. Line a baking sheet with baking paper.
- In a food processor, add the chia seed mixture and remaining ingredients and pulse for about 3 minutes.
- Place the bread mixture evenly in the prepared baking dish.
- Bake for about 1 1/2 hours or until a toothpick inserted into the center comes out clean.
- Remove the pan from the oven and place on a rack to cool for about 10 minutes.
- Carefully flip the loaf onto the rack to cool completely before slicing.
- Using a sharp knife, cut the loaf into desired size slices and serve.

Nutrition: Calories

16) Zucchini and banana bread

Preparation time: 15 minutes **Cooking time:** 45 minutes **Servings:** 6

Ingredients:
- ½ cup almond flour, sifted
- 1½ teaspoons of baking soda
- ½ teaspoon of cinnamon powder
- ¼ teaspoon ground cardamom

Ingredients:
- 1/8 teaspoon of clove powder
- 1½ cups banana, peeled and sliced
- ¼ cup almond butter, softened
- 2 teaspoons of organic vanilla extract
- 1 cup zucchini, shredded and squeezed

Directions:
- Preheat oven to 350 degrees F. Grease a 6x3-inch baking dish.
- In a large bowl, add the flour, baking soda and spices and with a fork, mix well.
- In another bowl, add the banana and use a fork to mash it completely.
- In the bowl of the banana, add the almond butter and vanilla extract and beat until well combined.
- Add the flour mixture and stir until just combined.
- Gently add the grated zucchini.
- Pour the flour mixture evenly into the prepared baking dish.
- Bake for about 40-45 minutes or until a toothpick inserted into the center comes out clean.
- Remove from the oven and place the pan on a wire rack to cool for at least 10 minutes.
- Carefully flip the bread onto the rack to cool completely before slicing.

Nutrition: Calories

17) *Granola with coconut, nuts and seeds*

Preparation time: 15 minutes   **Cooking time:** 23 minutes   **Servings:** 8

Ingredients:
- ½ cup unsweetened coconut flakes
- 1 cup raw almonds
- 1 cup raw walnuts
- ½ cup raw, shelled sunflower seeds
- ¼ cup of coconut oil

Directions:
- Preheat oven to 275 F. Line a large baking sheet with baking paper.
- In a food processor, add the coconut flakes, almonds, nuts and seeds and pulse until finely chopped.
- Meanwhile, in a medium nonstick skillet, add the oil, maple syrup and vanilla extract and cook for 3 minutes over medium-high heat, stirring constantly.
- Remove from heat and immediately stir into the nut mixture.
- Transfer the mixture to the prepared baking sheet and spread evenly.
- Cook for about 25 minutes, stirring twice.

Nutrition: Calories

Ingredients:
- ½ cup maple syrup
- 1 teaspoon of organic vanilla extract
- ½ cup golden raisins
- ½ cup of black raisins
- Sea salt, to taste
- Remove the pan from the oven and immediately stir in the raisins.
- Sprinkle with a little salt.
- With the back of a spatula, flatten the surface of the mixture.
- Set aside to cool completely.
- Next, break the granola into uniform sized pieces.
- Serve this granola with your choice of non-dairy milk and fruit toppings.
- To store, transfer this granola to an airtight container and store in the refrigerator.

18) *Tortilla Chips*

Preparation time: **Cooking time:** 30 minutes   **Servings:** 8

Ingredients:
- 2 cups of Spelt Flour
- 1 teaspoon of Pure Sea Salt

Directions:
- Set the oven to 350 degrees Fahrenheit.
- Place spelt flour and pure salt in a food processor*. Blend for about 15 seconds.
- While stirring, slowly add the soybean oil until well combined.
- Continue to blend and slowly add Spring Water to a dough is formed.
- Prepare a work surface and cover it with a piece of parchment paper. Sprinkle the flour on it.
- Knead the dough for about 1 to 2 minutes, until just right.
- Cover a baking pan with a little Grape Seed Oil.

Nutrition: Calories

Ingredients:
- 1/2 cup of rinse water
- 1/3 cup of ground olive oil
- Place the prepared dart in the baking dish.
- Brush the mixture with a little grape oil and, if desired, a little pure sea salt.
- Cut dough into 8 pieces with a pizza knife.
- Bake for about 10-12 minutes or until the chips are starting toecome golden brown.
- Allow to cool before serving.
- Serve and enjoy your Tortilla Chips!

Helpful Hints: If you don't have a refrigerator, you can use a hand mixer or blender. However, you will get better results with an immersion blender. You can serve the Tortillas with our Sweet Barbecue Sauce, Guacamole, or "Cheese". Sauce .

19) Onion Rings

Preparation time: **Cooking time:** 30 Minutes. **Servings:** 8

Ingredients:
- ✓ White onion or yellow onion
- ✓ 1 cup of Spelt Flour
- ✓ 1/2 cup of homemade Hempseed Milk
- ✓ 1/2 cup of Aquafaba *
- ✓ 2 teaspoons of Onion Powder.

Ingredients:
- ✓ 2 teaspoons of Oregano
- ✓ 1 teaspoon of Cayenne powder
- ✓ 2 teaspoons of Pure Sea Salt
- ✓ 3 tablespoons of grape oil

Directions:
- ❖ Preheat our oven to 450 degrees Fahrenheit.
- ❖ Pour Homemade Hempseed Milk and Aquafaba into a medium bowl and mix well.
- ❖ Add 1 teaspoon of Oregano, 1 teaspoon of Onion Powder, 1/2 teaspoon of Cayenne, and 1 teaspoon of Pure Sea Salt to the wet ingredients and mix.
- ❖ Peel the Onions, slice the ends.
- ❖ Cut peeled onion into slices about 1/4 inch thick. Cut the onion into rings.
- ❖ Add the Spelt flour, 1 teaspoon of Oregano, 1 teaspoon of Onion Powder, 1/2 teaspoon of Cayenne, and 1
- ❖ taspoon of Pure Sea Salt in a container with a quart. Shake out all the liquid.
- ❖ Brush a baking sheet with Grape Seed Oil 8. Place a couple onion rings over the water mixture.
- ❖ Put the water onion rings in the dry mixture and turn until coated on both sides.
- ❖ Place the covered onion rings on the baking sheet.
- ❖ Repeat steps 8 to 10 until all onion rings are covere.
- ❖ Lightly spray the rings with Grape seed oil.
- ❖ Water for about 10-15 minutes until it shines.
- ❖ This is all possible for coool them before serving.
- ❖ Serve and enjoy our onion rings!

Nutrition: Calories

Helpful Hints: If you haven't made Aquafaba, add 1/2 extra millet of Homemade hemp seed milk. You can use Onion rings with our sweet Bärbecue Sauce , or "Cheese" Sauce .

20) Strawberry Sorbet

Preparation time: 4 hours **Cooking time:** **Servings:** 4

Ingredients:
- ✓ 2 cups of Strawberries*.
- ✓ 1 1/2 teaspoons of spelt flour

Ingredients:
- ✓ 1/2 cup of sugar Date
- ✓ 2 cups of Spring Water

Directions:
- ❖ Add the sugar Date, water and flour Spelt in a saucepan and simmer for about ten minutes. The mixture should look like a syrup.
- ❖ Remove the meat from the cap and let it rest.
- ❖ After cooling, add Strawberry puree and stir.
- ❖ Place this mixture in a container and freeze.
- ❖ Cut it into pieces, put the butter in a bowl and beat until it reaches the limit.
- ❖ Place all the butter in the container and let it chill for at least four hours.
- ❖ Serve and enjoyy your Strawberry Sorbet!

Nutrition: Calories

Helpful hints: If you don't have fresh berries, you can use frozen ones.

Chapter 3 -   Lunch Recipes

21) Tomato and vegetable salad

Preparation time: 15 minutes. Cooking time: Servings: 4

Ingredients:
- ✓ 6 cups of fresh vegetables
- ✓ 2 cups of cherry tomatoes
- ✓ 2 shallots, chopped

Directions:
- ❖ Place all ingredients in a large bowl and mix to coat well.

Ingredients:
- ✓ 2 tablespoons of extra virgin olive oil
- ✓ 2 tablespoons fresh orange juice
- ✓ 1 tablespoon fresh lemon juice

- ❖ Cover the bowl and refrigerate for about 6-8 hours.
- ❖ Remove from refrigerator and mix well before serving.

Nutrition: Calories

22) Cauliflower Soup

Preparation time: 15 minutes Cooking time: 30 minutes. Servings: 4

Ingredients:
- ✓ 2 tablespoons of olive oil
- ✓ 1 yellow onion, chopped
- ✓ 2 carrots, peeled and cut into pieces
- ✓ 2 garlic cloves, minced
- ✓ 1 Serrano bell pepper, finely chopped
- ✓ 2 stalks of celery, chopped
- ✓ 1 teaspoon ground turmeric
- ✓ 1 teaspoon of ground coriander

Directions:
- ❖ Heat the oil over medium heat in a large soup pot and sauté the onion, carrot and celery for about 4-6 minutes.
- ❖ Add the garlic, serrano pepper and spices and sauté for about 1 minute.
- ❖ Add the cauliflower and cook for about 5 minutes, stirring occasionally.

Ingredients:
- ✓ 1 teaspoon of ground cumin
- ✓ ¼ teaspoon of red pepper flakes, crushed
- ✓ 1 head of cauliflower, chopped
- ✓ 4 cups of homemade vegetable broth
- ✓ 1 cup unsweetened coconut milk
- ✓ Sea salt and freshly ground black pepper, to taste
- ✓ 2 tablespoons fresh chives, finely chopped

- ❖ Add the broth and coconut milk and bring to a boil over medium-high heat.
- ❖ Reduce the heat to low and simmer for about 15 minutes.
- ❖ Season the soup with salt and black pepper and remove from heat.
- ❖ Using an immersion blender, blend the soup until smooth.
- ❖ Serve warm and garnish with chives.

Nutrition: Calories

23) Tomato Soup

Preparation time: 15 minutes   **Cooking time**: 45 minutes   **Servings**: 4

Ingredients:
- 2 tablespoons of coconut oil
- 2 carrots, coarsely chopped
- 1 large white onion, coarsely chopped
- 3 garlic cloves, minced
- 5 large tomatoes, coarsely chopped

Directions:
- Melt the coconut oil in a large soup pot over medium heat and cook the carrot and onion for about 10 minutes, stirring often.
- Add the garlic and sauté for about 1-2 minutes.
- Add the tomatoes, tomato paste, basil, broth, salt and black pepper and bring to a boil.

Nutrition: Calories

Ingredients:
- 1 tablespoon of homemade tomato paste
- 3 cups of homemade vegetable broth
- ¼ cup fresh basil, chopped
- ¼ cup unsweetened coconut milk
- Sea salt and freshly ground black pepper, to taste
- Reduce the heat to low and simmer uncovered for about 30 minutes.
- Add the coconut milk and remove from heat.
- Using an immersion blender, blend the soup until smooth.
- Serve hot.

24) Garlic broccoli

Preparation time: 10 minutes   **Cooking time**: 8 minutes   **Servings**: 2

Ingredients:
- 1 tablespoon of extra virgin olive oil
- 3-4 garlic cloves, minced

Directions:
- Heat the oil over medium heat in a large skillet and sauté the garlic for about 1 minute.
- Add the broccoli and sauté for about 2 minutes.

Nutrition: Calories

Ingredients:
- 2 cups of broccoli florets
- 2 tablespoons of tamari
- Add the tamari and sauté for about 4-5 minutes or until desired doneness.
- Remove from heat and serve hot.

25) Curried okra

Preparation time: 10 minutes   **Cooking time**: 15 minutes   **Servings**: 3

Ingredients:
- 1 tablespoon of olive oil
- ½ teaspoon of cumin seeds
- ¾ lb okra pods, trimmed and cut into 2-inch pieces
- ½ teaspoon of curry powder

Directions:
- Heat oil in a large skillet over medium heat
- For about 30 seconds, sauté the cumin seeds
- Add the okra and sauté for about 1-1½ minutes.
- Reduce heat to low and cook covered for about 6-8 minutes, stirring occasionally.

Nutrition: Calories

Ingredients:
- ½ teaspoon of chili powder
- 1 teaspoon of ground coriander
- Sea salt and freshly ground black pepper, to taste
- Add the curry powder, red pepper and cilantro and stir to combine.
- Increase the heat to medium and cook uncovered for another 2-3 minutes or so.
- Season with the salt and pepper and remove from heat.
- Serve hot.

26) Mushrooms curry

Preparation time: 20 minutes   **Cooking time**: 20 minutes   **Servings**: 4

Ingredients:
- 2 cups of tomatoes, chopped
- 1 green chili pepper, chopped
- 1 teaspoon fresh ginger, chopped
- 2 tablespoons of olive oil
- ½ teaspoon of cumin seeds
- ¼ teaspoon ground coriander
- ¼ teaspoon ground turmeric

Directions:
- In a food processor, add the tomatoes, green chiles and ginger and pulse until it forms a smooth paste.
- Heat the oil in a skillet over medium heat.
- For about 1 minute, sauté the cumin seeds.
- Add the spices and sauté for about 1 minute.

Nutrition: Calories

Ingredients:
- ¼ teaspoon of chili powder
- 2 cups fresh shiitake mushrooms, sliced
- 2 cups fresh button mushrooms, sliced
- 1¼ cup of water
- ¼ cup unsweetened coconut milk
- Sea salt and freshly ground black pepper, to taste

- Add the tomato mixture and cook for about 5 minutes.
- Add the mushrooms, water and coconut milk and bring to a boil.
- Cook for about 10-12 minutes, stirring occasionally.
- Season with the salt and black pepper and remove from heat.
- Serve hot.

27) Glazed Brussels sprouts

Preparation time: 15 minutes   **Cooking time**: 15 minutes   **Servings**: 3

Ingredients:
- 3 cups Brussels sprouts, cut and halved
- Sea salt, to taste
- 2 tablespoons of coconut oil, melted
- For the orange glaze:
- 1 tablespoon of coconut oil
- 2 small shallots, thinly sliced

Directions:
- Preheat oven to 400 degrees F. Line a baking sheet with baking paper.
- In a bowl, add the Brussels sprouts, a little salt and oil and toss to coat well.
- Transfer the mixture to the prepared baking dish.
- Roast for about 10-15 minutes, turning once halfway through.
- Meanwhile, prepare the frosting.
- In a skillet, melt the coconut oil over medium heat and sauté the scallions for about 5 minutes.
- Add the orange zest and sauté for about 1 minute.

Nutrition: Calories

Ingredients:
- 2 tablespoons of fresh orange zest, finely grated
- ¼ teaspoon ground ginger
- 2/3 cup fresh orange juice
- 1 tablespoon of sambal oelek (raw chili paste)
- 2 tablespoons of coconut amino acids
- 1 teaspoon of tapioca starch
- Sea salt, to taste
- Stir in the ginger, orange juice, sambal oelek and coconut amino acid and cook for about 5 minutes.
- Slowly add the tapioca starch, whisking constantly.
- Cook for about 2-3 minutes longer, stirring often.
- Add salt and remove from heat.
- Transfer roasted Brussels sprouts to a serving platter. Top evenly with the orange glaze.
- Serve immediately garnished with scallions.

28) Sauteed mushrooms

Preparation time: 15 minutes   **Cooking time**: 16 minutes   **Servings**: 2

Ingredients:
- 2 tablespoons of olive oil
- ½ teaspoon cumin seeds, lightly crushed
- 2 medium onions, thinly sliced

Directions:
- Heat oil in a frying pan over medium heat
- For about 1 minute, sauté the cumin seeds.
- Add the onion and sauté for about 4-5 minutes.

Nutrition: Calories

Ingredients:
- ¾ lb fresh mushrooms, chopped
- Sea salt and freshly ground black pepper, to taste

- Add the mushrooms and sauté for about 5-7 minutes.
- Add the salt and black pepper and sauté for about 2-3 minutes.
- Remove from heat and serve hot.

29) Sweet and sour cabbage

Preparation time: 10 minutes   **Cooking time:** 20 minutes   **Servings:** 4

Ingredients:
- 1 tablespoon of extra virgin olive oil
- 1 lemon, with seeds and thinly sliced
- 1 onion, chopped
- 3 garlic cloves, minced

Directions:
- In a large skillet, heat the oil over medium heat and cook the lemon slices for about 5 minutes.
- Using a slotted spoon, remove the lemon slices.

Ingredients:
- 2 pounds of fresh cabbage, hard ribs removed and trimmed
- ½ cup shallots, chopped
- 1 tablespoon of agave nectar
- Sea salt and freshly ground black pepper, to taste
- In the same skillet, add the onion and garlic and sauté for about 5 minutes.
- Add the cabbage, scallions, agave nectar, salt and black pepper and cook for about 8-10 minutes, stirring occasionally.
- Remove from heat and serve hot.

Nutrition: Calories

30) Brussels sprouts with walnuts

Preparation time: 15 minutes   **Cooking time:** 15 minutes   **Servings:** 2

Ingredients:
- ½ pound Brussels sprouts, halved
- 1 tablespoon of olive oil
- 2 garlic cloves, minced
- ½ teaspoon of red pepper flakes, crushed

Directions:
- Place a steamer basket in a large pot of boiling water.
- Place Brussels sprouts in the basket of the steamer and steam, covered for about 6-8 minutes.
- Drain Brussels sprouts well.
- In a large skillet, heat the oil over medium heat and sauté the garlic and red pepper flakes for about 40 seconds.

Ingredients:
- Sea salt and freshly ground black pepper, to taste
- 1 tablespoon fresh lemon juice
- 1 tablespoon pine nuts

- Add the Brussels sprouts, salt and black pepper and sauté for about 4-5 minutes.
- Add the lemon juice and sauté for about 1 minute more.
- Add pine nuts and remove from heat.
- Serve hot.

Nutrition: Calories

31) Roasted Butternut Squash

Preparation time: 15 minutes   **Cooking time:** 45 minutes   **Servings:** 6

Ingredients:
- 8 cups butternut squash, peeled, seeded and diced
- 2 tablespoons of melted almond butter
- ½ teaspoon ground cinnamon

Directions:
- Preheat oven to 425 degrees F. Place foil pieces on 2 baking sheets.
- In a large bowl, add all ingredients and mix to coat well.

Ingredients:
- ½ teaspoon of ground cumin
- ¼ teaspoon of red pepper flakes
- Sea salt, to taste

- Arrange the pumpkin pieces on the prepared baking sheets in a single layer.
- Roast for about 40-45 minutes.
- Remove from oven and serve.

Nutrition: Calories

32) Broccoli with peppers

Preparation time: 15 minutes   **Cooking time:** 10 minutes   **Servings:** 4

Ingredients:
- 2 tablespoons of olive oil
- 4 garlic cloves, minced
- 1 large white onion, sliced
- 2 cups of small broccoli florets

Directions:
- In a large skillet, heat the oil over medium heat and sauté the garlic for about 1 minute.

Ingredients:
- 3 red peppers, seeded and sliced
- ¼ cup homemade vegetable broth
- Sea salt and freshly ground black pepper, to taste

- Add the onion, broccoli and peppers and sauté for about 5 minutes.
- Add the broth and sauté for about 4 more minutes.
- Serve hot.

33) Shrimp with tamari

Preparation time: 15 minutes   **Cooking time:** 6 minutes   **Servings:** 2

Ingredients:
- ✓ 1 tablespoon of olive oil
- ✓ 2 garlic cloves, minced
- ✓ ½ pound of raw, peeled and deveined jumbo shrimps

Directions:
- ❖ In a large skillet, heat the oil over medium heat and sauté the garlic for about 1 minute.

Nutrition: Calories

Ingredients:
- ✓ 2 tablespoons of tamari
- ✓ Freshly ground black pepper, to taste

- ❖ Stir in the shrimp, tamari and black pepper and cook for about 4-5 minutes or until completely done.
- ❖ Serve hot.

34) Vegetarian Kebab

Preparation time: 20 minutes **Cooking time:** 10 minutes **Servings:** 4

Ingredients:
- For the marinade:
- ✓ 2 garlic cloves, minced
- ✓ 2 teaspoons fresh basil, chopped
- ✓ 2 teaspoons fresh oregano, chopped
- ✓ ½ teaspoon of cayenne pepper
- ✓ Sea salt and freshly ground black pepper, to taste
- ✓ 2 tablespoons fresh lemon juice

Directions:
- ❖ For the marinade: in a large bowl, add all ingredients and mix until well combined.
- ❖ Add the vegetables to the marinade and toss to coat well.
- ❖ Cover and refrigerate to marinate the vegetables for at least 6-8 hours.
- ❖ In a large bowl of water, soak the wooden skewers for at least 30 minutes.

Nutrition: Calories

Ingredients:
- ✓ 2 tablespoons of olive oil
- For vegetables:
- ✓ 2 large zucchini, cut into thick slices
- ✓ 8 large button mushrooms, quartered
- ✓ 1 yellow bell pepper, seeded and diced
- ✓ 1 red bell pepper, seeded and diced

- ❖ Preheat grill to medium-high heat. Generously grease the grill grate.
- ❖ Remove the vegetables from the bowl and discard the marinade.
- ❖ Thread the vegetables onto the pre-soaked wooden skewers, starting with the zucchini, mushrooms and peppers.
- ❖ Grill for about 8-10 minutes or until cooked through, turning occasionally.

35) Fried onion sprout

Preparation time: 5 minutes **Cooking time:** 10 minutes **Servings:** 4

Ingredients:
- ✓ 2½ pounds Brussels sprouts, cut4 slices bacon, cut into 1-inch pieces
- ✓ 1 tablespoon of extra virgin coconut oil
- ✓ 1 tomato, chopped
- ✓ 1 onion, chopped

Directions:
- ❖ Add sprouts to boiling water in a pot.
- ❖ Let them cook for about 3-5 minutes.
- ❖ Drain and set aside.
- ❖ Saute onions in a greased skillet for 4 minutes.

Nutrition: Calories

Ingredients:
- ✓ 4 sprigs of thyme or savory, divided
- ✓ 1 teaspoon celtic sea salt, iodine-free
- ✓ Freshly ground pepper to taste
- ✓ 2 teaspoons of lemon juice (optional)

- ❖ Mix with salt, pepper and thyme
- ❖ Add the drained sprouts to the skillet and stir for 3 minutes.
- ❖ Remove and discard sprigs of grasses.
- ❖ Serve warm with lemon juice and chopped spring onion on top.

36) Southwestern stuffed sweet potatoes

Preparation time: Cooking time: Portions:

Ingredients:
- ✓ Sliced avocado (1)
- ✓ Pinch of cumin
- ✓ Pinch of dried red chili flakes
- ✓ Spinach (3 c.)
- ✓ Sliced shallot (1)
- ✓ Black beans (.5 c.)
- ✓ Coconut oil (2 tablespoons)
- ✓ Sweet potatoes

Ingredients:
- ✓ Drugs
- ✓ Pepper and salt
- ✓ Chopped coriander (1 handful)
- ✓ Cumin (1 teaspoon)
- ✓ Lime Juice (1)
- ✓ Olive oil (3 tablespoons)

Directions:
- ❖ Turn on the oven and give it time to heat up to 400 degrees. Clean the sweet potatoes and pierce them a few times with a fork.
- ❖ Add baking paper to a baking sheet and place sweet potatoes on top. Add to the oven to bake.
- ❖ After 50 minutes, the potatoes should be soft. Remove them from the oven and give them time to cool.
- ❖ Meanwhile, take a skillet and add the coconut oil along with the black beans and shallots.
- ❖ Cook these for a few minutes before adding the cumin, chili flakes and spinach, stirring to mix well.
- ❖ Finally, take a small bowl and whisk the ingredients for the dressing well.
- ❖ Cut the sweet potatoes in half before stuffing them with the black bean mixture you made.
- ❖ Add a few slices of avocado and some of the dressing poured over before serving.

Nutrition: Calories

37) Zoodles with cream sauce

Preparation time: Cooking time: Portions:

Ingredients:
- ✓ Toasted pepitas (2 tablespoons)
- ✓ Pepper (.5 tsp.)
- ✓ Salt (1 teaspoon)
- ✓ Chopped coriander (2 tablespoons)
- ✓ Water (1 tablespoon)

Ingredients:
- ✓ Lemon juice (.5)
- ✓ Olive oil (2 tablespoons)
- ✓ Pitted avocado (1)
- ✓ Spiral zucchini (1)
- ✓ Coconut oil (1 tablespoon)

Directions:
- ❖ Add a little coconut oil to melt in a skillet before adding the zucchini noodles. Cook for 5 minutes before turning off the heat.
- ❖ Take out a blender and combine together the pepper, salt, 1 tablespoon cilantro, water, lemon juice, oil and avocado. Mix well and cook to make the cream.
- ❖ Add the sauce to the skillet with the noodles and stir to combine. Move to a serving bowl and add the rest of the cilantro and toasted pepitas before serving.

Nutrition: Calories

38) Rainbow Pad Thai

Preparation time: Cooking time: Portions:

Ingredients:
- ✓ Avocado cubes (1)
- ✓ Chopped coriander (1 c.)
- ✓ Shredded daikon radish (1 c.)
- ✓ Chopped broccoli (1 c.)
- ✓ Shredded red cabbage (1 c.)
- ✓ Sliced shallots (3)
- ✓ Shredded carrots (2)
- ✓ Spiral Zucchini (3)

Ingredients:
- For the dressing
- ✓ Chopped ginger (1 teaspoon)
- ✓ Chopped garlic clove (1)
- ✓ Sesame oil (1 tablespoon)
- ✓ Tahini (.25 c.)
- ✓ Lime Juice (1)

Directions:
- ❖ Add ingredients for Pad Thai, except avocado, to a large bowl and mix.
- ❖ Blend together all the ingredients you have for the dressing until creamy and combined.
- ❖ Top the vegetables with the diced avocado and pour the dressing over them before serving.

Nutrition: Calories

39) Lentils and vegetables

Preparation time: Cooking time: Portions:

Ingredients:
- ✓ Avocado (1)
- ✓ Crushed almonds (1 tablespoon)
- ✓ Crushed black pepper (1 teaspoon)
- ✓ Salt (1 teaspoon)
- ✓ Arugula (1 c.)

Ingredients:
- ✓ Cooked wild rice (1 c.)
- ✓ Lemon juice (.5)
- ✓ Diced Carrot (1)
- ✓ Broccoli florets (.5 c.)
- ✓ Sliced Pak choi (.5 c.)

- ✓ Brown or green lentils (.5 c.)
- ✓ Vegetable stock (.25 c.)

Directions:
- ❖ Add the vegetable broth to a skillet over medium heat. Let it begin to simmer before adding the lemon juice, carrot, broccoli and pak choi.
- ❖ After 5 minutes, turn off the heat and stir in the almonds, pepper, salt, arugula, lentils and wild rice.
- ❖ Move this mixture to plates and top with a few slices of avocado before serving.

Nutrition: Calories

40) Vegetable dish with sesame

Preparation time: Cooking time: Portions:

Ingredients:
- ✓ Sesame seeds (1 teaspoon)
- ✓ Lemon juice (.5)
- ✓ Tamari Sauce (2 tablespoons)
- ✓ Chopped garlic clove (1)
- ✓ Diced red bell pepper (.5 c.)

Ingredients:
- ✓ Finely chopped broccoli florets (2 c.)
- ✓ Cubed tofu (8 ounces)
- ✓ Olive oil (2 tablespoons)
- ✓ Sesame oil, toasted (1.5 tablespoons)

Directions:
- ❖ Heat half a tablespoon of sesame oil and one tablespoon of olive oil in a skillet. Add the tofu and let it cook for a bit.
- ❖ After ten minutes, remove the tofu and add a little more of the two oils.
- ❖ Stir in the garlic, red bell bell pepper and broccoli until they soften a bit. Add the tofu and stir in the lemon juice and soy sauce as well.
- ❖ Top this dish with a few sesame seeds before serving.

Nutrition: Calories

Chapter 4 -   Dinner Recipes

41) Stew without beef

Preparation time: Cooking time: Servings: 4

Ingredients:
- Dried oregano, 1 teaspoon
- Celery, diced, 2 stalks
- Large diced potato
- Sliced carrot, 3 c.
- Water, 2 c.
- Vegetable broth, 3 c.

Ingredients:
- Pepper, one teaspoon
- Sea salt, one teaspoon
- Garlic puree, 2 bulbs
- Diced onion, 1 c.
- Avocado oil, 1 tablespoon
- Laurel

Directions:
- Heat the avocado oil in a top pan. Put in the pepper, salt, garlic cloves and onion bulbs. Cook everything for two to three minutes, or until the onion is soft.
- Add the bay leaf, oregano, celery, potato, carrot, water and broth. Allow to simmer, then lower the heat and prepare for 30-45 minutes, or until the carrots and potatoes become soft.
- Taste and adjust seasonings as needed. If it's too thick, you can add more water or broth.
- Divide among four bowls and enjoy.

Nutrition: Calories

42) Emmenthal soup

Preparation time: Cooking time: Servings: 2

Ingredients:
- Cayenne
- Nutmeg
- Pumpkin seeds, 1 tablespoon
- Chopped chives, 2 tablespoons

Ingredients:
- Diced Emmenthal cheese, 3 tablespoons
- Vegetable broth, 2 c.
- Diced potato, 1
- Shredded cauliflower, 2 c.

Directions:
- Place the potato and cauliflower in a saucepan with the vegetable broth until tender.
- Place in a blender and blend.
- Add the spices and adjust to taste.
- Pour into bowls, add chives and cheese and mix well.
- Garnish with pumpkin seeds. Enjoy.

Nutrition: Calories

43) Spaghetti with broccoli

Preparation time: Cooking time: Servings: 2

Ingredients:
- Pepper
- Halls
- Vegetable broth, 1 teaspoon
- Oregano plant, 1 teaspoon
- Lemon juice, 1 tablespoon
- Sliced carrots, 3
- Diced tomatoes, 3

Ingredients:
- Broccoli cut into florets, 1 head
- Sliced red bell pepper - bell, one
- Sliced onion bulb, one
- Diced garlic bulbs, two cloves
- EVOO, 4 tablespoons
- Buckwheat pasta, 1 lb.

Directions:
- Place a pot of water halfway up and add the salt. Allow to boil and add the pasta. Prepare according to box instructions. Empty.
- Place broccoli in another bowl and cover with h2O. Prepare for five minutes.
- Place a skillet over normal heat and put two tablespoons of olive oil in the pan and heat. Place the bulbs, garlic and onion in and prepare until soft and fragrant. Remove from the skillet and set aside.
- carrots. Cook for five minutes, then put in the sweet bell pepper and prepare for another five minutes, now put in the tomatoes and prepare for two minutes.
- Drain the broccoli completely and add it to the skillet with the rest of the vegetables. Return the onions and garlic to the skillet.
- Add the vegetable broth, oregano and lemon juice. Add a little pepper and salt, taste and adjust seasonings if needed. Stir well to combine.
- Place the cooked pasta on a serving plate. Pour over the vegetable mixture and toss to combine.

Nutrition: Calories

44) Indian Lentil Curry

Preparation time: Cooking time: Servings: 4 - 6

Ingredients:
- ✓ Lime Juice
- ✓ Chopped coriander
- ✓ Halls
- ✓ EVOO, 1 tablespoon
- ✓ Diced tomatoes, 2
- ✓ Sliced onion, 1

Directions:
- ❖ Place lentils in a bowl, cover with water and let stand for six hours.
- ❖ After six hours, drain the lentils completely.
- ❖ Place a bowl over normal heat. Place lentils and cover with fresh water. Allow to boil. Add turmeric. Lower heat and simmer until lentils are cooked.
- ❖ Remove from the pan and place in a bowl. Set aside.

Nutrition: Calories

Ingredients:
- ✓ Chopped garlic, 1 clove
- ✓ Grated ginger, 1 inch
- ✓ Turmeric, .5 tsp
- ✓ Cumin seeds, .5 tsp
- ✓ Chopped green peppers, 2
- ✓ Fine red lentils, 1 c.
- ❖ In another skillet over medium heat, heat the olive oil. Add the turmeric, cumin, ginger and onions. Cook until the onions are soft and the ginger is fragrant.
- ❖ Add the chiles and tomatoes and cook. Add the salt and cook for five minutes.
- ❖ Pour the lentil into this mixture and bring back to a simmer. As soon as it starts to cook, remove it from the hot temperature. Squeeze a little lemon
- ❖ Sprinkle with cilantro and serve with rice.

45) Vegetables with wild rice

Preparation time: Cooking time: Servings: 4

Ingredients:
- ✓ Halls
- ✓ Basil
- ✓ Cilantro
- ✓ Juice of a lime
- ✓ Chopped red bell pepper, 1
- ✓ Vegetable broth, .5 c.

Directions:
- ❖ Place all the chopped vegetables in a pan and add the vegetable broth.
- ❖ Steam fry the vegetables until cooked but still crispy.

Nutrition: Calories

Ingredients:
- ✓ Bean sprouts, 1 c.
- ✓ Chopped carrots, 2 c.
- ✓ Beans - green - diced, 1 c.
- ✓ Broccoli, cut, 1 c.
- ✓ Pak Choi, 1 c.
- ✓ Wild rice, 1 c.
- ❖ Using a mortar and pestle, grind the chili, basil, and cilantro until they form a paste. Add the lime juice and mix well.
- ❖ Place the rice on a serving plate. Add the vegetables on top and drizzle with the dressing.

46) Spicy Lentil Soup

Preparation time: Cooking time: Servings: 4

Ingredients:
- ✓ Halls
- ✓ Turmeric, .25 tsp
- ✓ Chopped garlic, 3 cloves
- ✓ Grated ginger, 1.5 inch piece
- ✓ Chopped tomato, 1

Directions:
- ❖ Place lentils in a colander and place under running water. Rinse until the soil and stones are released.
- ❖ Pour rinsed lentils into a pot. Add enough water to cover the lentils. Place the pot over medium heat and allow to boil.

Nutrition: Calories

Ingredients:
- ✓ Chopped Serrano chili pepper, 1
- ✓ Rinsed red lentils, 2 c.
- ✓ Topping:
- ✓ Coconut yogurt, .25 c.
- ❖ Lower the heat and simmer for ten minutes.
- ❖ Place the contents of the leftovers and then mix well to combine.
- ❖ Cook again until lentils are soft.
- ❖ Garnish with a spoonful of coconut yogurt.

47) Leek soup with mushrooms

Preparation time: Cooking time: Servings: 4

Ingredients:
- Sherry vinegar, 1.5 tablespoons
- Almond milk, .5 c.
- Cream of coconut, .66 c.
- Vegetable broth, 3 c.
- Chopped dill, 1 tablespoon
- Pepper
- Halls

Directions:
- Set a Dutch oven to medium and heat the oil. Add the leeks and bulb garlic and prepare until soft.
- Add the mushrooms, stir and cook for another 10 minutes.

Nutrition: Calories

Ingredients:
- Almond flour, 5 tablespoons
- Cleaned and sliced mushrooms, 7 c.
- Chopped garlic, 3 cloves
- Chopped leeks, 2.75 c.
- Vegetable oil, 3 tablespoons

- Add the salt, dill, pepper and flour. Mix well, until combined.
- Put the soup in and let it simmer. Reduce the heat and put in the rest of the ingredients. Stir well. Cook another ten minutes.
- Serve hot with almond flour bread.

48) Fresh vegetarian pizza

Preparation time: Cooking time: Servings: 4

Ingredients:
- Crust -
- Garlic bulb flavored powder, 0.5 teaspoon
- Sea salt, 0.5 teaspoon
- Coconut oil, 3 tablespoons
- Almond flour, 1.25 c.
- Tahini-Bee Spread -
- Pepper, pinch

Directions:
- Start by setting your oven to 375. Place some parchment on a tray.
- Mix together the salt, garlic powder, coconut oil and almond flour.
- Place it on the tray and squish it into a ball shape. Place another piece of parchment on top and roll out the dough into a 7x7 square. Bake for 14 minutes, or until it starts to brown.

Nutrition: Calories

Ingredients:
- Sea salt, a pinch
- Garlic, 2 cloves
- Lemon juice, one tablespoon
- Avocado oil, one tablespoon
- Middle Eastern Pasta, one tablespoon
- Peeled and diced beets, 2

- While the crust is cooking, add the pepper, salt, garlic, lemon juice, avocado oil, tahini, and beets to a food processor. Blend until creamy.
- To make your pizza, spread the crust with beet sauces and then top with your favorite alkaline friendly vegetables. Cut it into four and enjoy.

49) Spicy Lentil Burger

Preparation time: Cooking time: Servings: 4

Ingredients:
- Avocado oil, 1 tablespoon
- Coconut flour, 1 tablespoon
- Crushed garlic, 2 cloves
- Jalapeno cubes
- Chopped cilantro, .5 c.

Directions:
- Cook lentils according to package instructions and set aside to cool.
- Mix together the garlic, jalapeno, cilantro, onion, pepper, salt, almond meal and lentils until everything is well combined.
- Add half of the lentil mixture to a food processor and process until it reaches a paste-like consistency.
- Pour this into the bowl with the rest of the lentil mixture and toss to combine.

Nutrition: Calories

Ingredients:
- Diced onion, .5 c.
- Pepper, .5 tsp
- Sea salt, 0.5 teaspoons
- Almond flour, .5 c.
- Dried lentils, .5 c.

- The mixture will be very moist. Stir in the coconut flour to help get rid of the moisture and to help hold them together.
- Divide the mixture into quarters. Squeeze a quarter of the mixture between your hands to flatten it into a hamburger shape. Do this for the remaining three sections.
- Heat the oil in a large skillet and place the burgers in it. Prepare the burgers 4 to 6 minutes on both sides, or until golden brown. When you flip them, do so carefully so they don't fall apart. Enjoy.

50) Roasted cauliflower rolls

Preparation time: Cooking time: Servings: 2

Ingredients:
- Cauliflower -
- Pepper, .25 tsp
- Sea salt, .25 tsp
- Garlic powder, .5 tsp
- Nutritional yeast, .25 c.
- Almond flour, .25 c.
- Avocado oil, 1 tablespoon
- Bitten cauliflower florets, 2 c.
- Sauce -
- Sea Salt

Ingredients:
- Apple cider vinegar, 2 tablespoons
- Garlic, 2 cloves
- Habanero Pepper
- Mango cubes, 1 c.
- Assembly -
- Canola shoots, 2 leaves
- Mixed salad, 1 c.

Directions:
- Start by setting your kitchen appliance to three hundred and fifty degrees then place paper on a kitchen wrap.
- To prepare the cauliflower, toss it in the avocado oil and make sure it's evenly coated.
- In a container, combine together all the seasonings: pepper, salt, garlic powder, healthy mushrooms, along with almond flour.
- Sprinkle breading over cauliflower and toss, making sure cauliflower is well coated. Spread on the baking sheet.

- Bake thirty to thirty-five minutes, or until cauliflower is soft.
- While the cauliflower is cooking, add the salt, vinegar, garlic, habanero and mango to your blender and blend until well combined. Be sure to use gloves or wash your hands thoroughly when you need to handle the habanero.
- To assemble, divide the salad mix between the collard leaves, top with the cauliflower and pour the sauce over it. Wrap the whole thing like a burrito and enjoy.

Nutrition: Calories

51) Sliced sweet potato with artichoke cream and peppers

Preparation time: Cooking time: Servings: 4

Ingredients:
- Pepper, .25 tsp
- Salt, .5 tsp
- Avocado oil, 6 tablespoons - divided
- Red bell pepper cut into quarters

Ingredients:
- Unpeeled sweet potatoes, 2 cut into 4 slices lengthwise
- Garlic, 2 cloves
- Artichoke hearts, 14 oz can

Directions:
- Start by setting the oven to 350. Place parchment on a tray and set aside.
- Spread the bell bell pepper and sweet potato on the sheet tray and top with two teaspoons of avocado oil, a pinch of pepper and a pinch of salt.

- Bake for 30 minutes. Turn them over and bake for another 15 minutes.
- Add the roasted red bell pepper to a food processor along with the garlic, artichoke hearts, pepper, salt and remaining avocado oil. Pulse until combined but still somewhat chunky. Adjust seasonings as needed.
- Top the sweet potato slices with the cream and enjoy.

Nutrition: Calories

52) Cooking scallops, onions and potatoes

Preparation time: Cooking time: Servings: 4

Ingredients:
- Cashew cheese sauce -
- Sea salt, 0.5 teaspoons
- Nutritional yeast, .5 c.
- Almond milk, 1 c.
- Raw cashews, 1 c.
- Scallop Bake -
- Chopped tarragon, 1 tablespoon

Directions:
- To make the cheese sauce, add the cashews to a bowl and cover them with room temperature water. Let them soak for 15-20 minutes and then drain and rinse them.
- Blend together cashews with remaining cheese sauce ingredients until smooth and creamy. Set aside until later.
- Start by heating the oven to 375.
- Combine the onions and potatoes in a bowl with the avocado oil. Add the tarragon, pepper and salt, making sure everything is well coated.

Nutrition: Calories

Ingredients:
- Pepper, 1 teaspoon
- Sea salt, one teaspoon
- Oil - Avocado, one tablespoon
- Chopped small onion bulbs, 1.5
- New potatoes, thinly sliced, 8

- Using an 8-inch square baking dish, place the potato and onion mixture in the dish. Do your best to arrange them in nice rows. It doesn't have to be perfect.
- Bake for 45 minutes, or until potatoes are soft
- Remove from oven and top with cheese sauce. Divide among four plates and enjoy. You can also slide this on, and bake inside the cooking appliance on about 5 minutes in order to warm the cheese sauce through before serving.

53) Spicy cilantro and coconut soup

Preparation time: Cooking time: Servings: 2

Ingredients:
- Cilantro leaves, 2 tablespoons
- Jalapeno
- Lime juice, 1 tablespoon
- Whole Coconut Milk, 13.5 oz. can

Directions:
- Add the avocado oil to a medium skillet and heat. Add the salt, garlic and onion, cooking three to five minutes, or until the onion bulbs become smooth.

Nutrition: Calories

Ingredients:
- Sea salt, .25 tsp
- Crushed garlic, 3 cloves
- Diced onion, .5 c.
- Avocado oil, 2 tablespoons
- Place the onion mixture, cilantro, jalapeno, lime juice and coconut milk in a blender and blend until creamy.
- Pour into a bowl and enjoy.

54) Tarragon soup

Preparation time: Cooking time: Servings: 2

Ingredients:
- Chopped fresh tarragon, 2 tablespoons
- Celery stalk
- Raw cashews, .5 c.
- Lemon juice, 1 tablespoon
- Whole Coconut Milk, 13.5 oz. can

Directions:
- Add the oil to a medium skillet and heat it up. Put all the seasonings: pepper, salt, garlic bulbs, along with the onion bulbs then prepare about three to five minutes, or until the onions become soft.

Nutrition: Calories

Ingredients:
- Pepper, .5 tsp - divided
- Sea Salt, .5 tsp - divided
- Crushed garlic, 3 cloves
- Diced onion, .5 c.
- Avocado oil, 1 tablespoon
- Using a high-speed blender, add the onion mixture, tarragon, celery, cashews, lemon juice, and coconut milk. Blend until smooth. Taste and adjust seasonings if necessary.
- Divide between two bowls and enjoy. You can also add back into a pot and reheat before serving.

55) Asparagus and artichoke soup

Preparation time: Cooking time: Servings: 4

Ingredients:
- ✓ Artichoke hearts halved and chopped, 1 can
- ✓ Almond milk, 2 c.
- ✓ Pepper, .5 tsp
- ✓ Sea Salt, .5 - .75 tsp
- ✓ Vegetable broth, 2 c.
- ✓ Asparagus diced, 8 stalks

Directions:
- ❖ Add the garlic, avocado oil and onion to a skillet and cook for a few minutes, or until the onion bulbs have softened and weakened.
- ❖ Place the cooked vegetables in a pot and add the pepper, salt, vegetable stock, asparagus and potatoes. Stir everything together and let it simmer. Lower the heat and simmer gently eighteen to twenty minutes, or until the potatoes have become soft.

Nutrition: Calories

Ingredients:
- ✓ Cubed potatoes, 1 c.
- ✓ Crushed garlic, 2 cloves
- ✓ Avocado oil, 1 tablespoon
- ✓ Diced onion, .5 c.

- ❖ Add a little more broth if you need it, so that the liquid remains about an inch above the vegetables.
- ❖ Set the pot away from the heat and let it cool.
- ❖ Using a blender, blend the cooled soup with the artichokes and almond milk until everything is well combined and smooth. Adjust seasonings as needed. You can add more broth or milk to thicken everything if needed.
- ❖ Pour back into the pot and allow to heat over low heat until ready to serve.

56) Mint and berry soup

Preparation time: Cooking time: Servings: 1

Ingredients:
- ✓ Sweetener -
- ✓ Water, .25 c - more if needed
- ✓ Unrefined whole cane sugar, .25 c.
- Soup -
- ✓ Water, .5 c.

Directions:
- ❖ Add the water and sugar to a small saucepan and cook, stirring constantly, until the sugar has dissolved. Allow to cool.
- ❖ Add the mint leaves, lemon juice, water, berries and cooled sugar mixture to a blender. Blend everything until smooth.

Nutrition: Calories

Ingredients:
- ✓ Mixed berries, 1 c.
- ✓ Mint leaves, 8
- ✓ Lemon juice, 1 teaspoon

- ❖ Pour into a bowl and then refrigerate until the broth is completely cooled. This will take about 20 minutes.
- ❖ Enjoy.

57) Mushroom soup

Preparation time: Cooking time: Servings: 2

Ingredients:
- ✓ Whole Coconut Milk, 13.5 oz. can
- ✓ Vegetable stock, 1 c.
- ✓ Pepper, .5 tsp
- ✓ Sea salt, .75 tsp
- ✓ Crush the garlic clove
- ✓ Diced onion, 1 cup

Directions:
- ❖ Heat the fat in a very massive pan, then put all the seasonings: pepper, salt, garlic, onion bulb and mushrooms. Boil and prepare for a few minutes, or until onions are soft.
- ❖ Stir in the coconut amino acid, thyme, coconut milk and vegetable broth.

Nutrition: Calories

Ingredients:
- ✓ Cut cremini mushrooms, 1 cup
- ✓ Chinese black mushrooms cut into pieces, one cup
- ✓ Avocado oil, 1 tablespoon
- ✓ Coconut amino acids, 1 tablespoon
- ✓ Dried thyme, .5 tsp

- ❖ Lower the heat and let the broth simmer for about fifteen minutes. Stir the broth occasionally.
- ❖ Taste and adjust seasoning as needed. Divide between two bowls and enjoy.

58) Potato and lentil stew

Preparation time: Cooking time: Servings: 4

Ingredients:
- Chopped oregano sprigs, 2 sprigs
- Diced celery stalk
- Potato diced and peeled, 1 c.
- Sliced carrots, 2
- Dried lentils, 1 c.
- Spicy seasoning / Pepper, one teaspoon
- Sea salt, one to 1.5 teaspoons

Directions:
- Using a large cooking utensil, heat the avocado fat along with the inclusion of seasonings: pepper, salt, garlic bulbs, along with the onion. Cook three to five minutes, or until onion is soft.
- Add the tarragon, oregano, celery, potato, carrots, lentils and 2 ½ cups of vegetable stock. Stir everything together.

Nutrition: Calories

Ingredients:
- Crushed garlic bulbs, two buds
- Diced onion, .5 c.
- Avocado oil, 2 tablespoons
- Whole Coconut Milk, 13.5 oz. can
- Vegetable broth, 5 c - divided
- Chopped tarragon, 2 sprigs

- Allow the saucepan to heat back up and then lower the heat. Allow to cook, stirring frequently. Add more vegetable broth in half-cup portions, if necessary, to make sure the lentils have enough liquid to cook. Let the stew cook for 20-25 minutes, or until the lentils and potatoes are soft.
- Remove stew from heat and stir in coconut milk. Divide among four bowls and enjoy.

59) Mixed mushroom stew

Preparation time: 15 minutes Cooking time: 15 minutes Servings: 4

Ingredients:
- 2 tablespoons of olive oil
- 2 onions, chopped
- 3 garlic cloves, minced
- ½ pound fresh mushrooms, chopped
- ¼ pound fresh shiitake mushrooms, chopped

Directions:
- In a large skillet, heat the oil over medium heat and sauté the onion and garlic for 4-5 minutes.
- Add the mushrooms, salt and black pepper and cook for 4-5 minutes.

Nutrition: Calories

Ingredients:
- ¼ pound fresh Portobello mushrooms, chopped
- Sea salt and freshly ground black pepper, to taste
- ¼ cup homemade vegetable broth
- ½ cup unsweetened coconut milk
- 2 tablespoons fresh parsley, chopped
- Add the broth and coconut milk and bring to a gentle boil.
- Simmer for 4-5 minutes or until desired doneness.
- Add the parsley and remove from heat.
- Serve warm.

60) Mixed stew of spicy vegetables

Preparation time: 20 minutes Cooking time: 35 minutes Servings: 8

Ingredients:
- 2 tablespoons of coconut oil
- 1 large sweet onion, chopped
- 1 medium parsnip, peeled and chopped
- 3 tablespoons of homemade tomato paste
- 2 large garlic cloves, minced
- ½ teaspoon of cinnamon powder
- ½ teaspoon ground ginger
- 1 teaspoon of ground cumin
- ¼ teaspoon cayenne pepper

Directions:
- In a large soup pot, melt the coconut oil over medium-high heat and sauté the onion for about 5 minutes.
- Add the parsnips and sauté for about 3 minutes.
- Add the tomato paste, garlic and spices and sauté for 2 minutes.

Nutrition: Calories

Ingredients:
- 2 medium carrots, peeled and chopped
- 2 medium purple potatoes, peeled and cut into pieces
- 2 medium sweet potatoes, peeled and cut into pieces
- 4 cups of homemade vegetable broth
- 2 tablespoons fresh lemon juice
- 2 cups fresh cabbage, hard ribs removed and chopped
- ¼ cup fresh parsley leaves, chopped

- Stir in the carrots, potatoes, sweet potatoes and broth and bring to a boil.
- Reduce heat to medium-low and simmer, covered for about 20 minutes.
- Add the lemon juice and cabbage and simmer for 5 minutes.
- Serve with a garnish of parsley.

Chapter 5 - Snacks Recipes

61) Bean burgers

Preparation time: 20 minutes **Cooking time:** 25 minutes **Servings:** 8

Ingredients:
- ½ cup of walnuts
- 1 carrot, peeled and chopped
- 1 celery stalk, chopped
- 4 shallots, chopped
- 5 cloves of garlic, minced

Directions:
- Preheat oven to 400 degrees F. Line a baking sheet with baking paper.
- In a food processor, add the walnuts and pulse until finely combined.
- Add the carrot, celery, shallot and garlic and run through a meat grinder until finely chopped.
- Transfer the vegetable mixture to a large bowl.
- In the same food processor, add the beans and pulse until chopped.

Nutrition: Calories

Ingredients:
- 2¼ cups canned black beans, rinsed and drained
- 2½ cups sweet potato, peeled and grated
- ½ teaspoon of red pepper flakes, crushed
- ¼ teaspoon cayenne pepper
- Sea salt and freshly ground black pepper, to taste

- Add 1 1/2 cups sweet potatoes and pulse until a chunky mixture forms.
- Transfer the bean mixture to the bowl with the vegetable mixture.
- Stir in remaining sweet potato and spices and mix until well combined.
- Make 8 equal-sized patties from the dough.
- Arrange the meatballs on the prepared baking sheet in a single layer.
- Bake for about 25 minutes.
- Serve hot.

62) Grilled watermelon

Preparation time: 10 minutes **Cooking time:** 4 minutes **Servings:** 4

Ingredients:
- 1 watermelon, peeled and cut into 1 inch thick wedges
- 1 garlic clove, finely chopped
- 2 tablespoons fresh lime juice

Directions:
- Preheat the grill to high heat. Grease the grill grate.
- Grill the watermelon pieces for about 2 minutes on both sides.

Nutrition: Calories

Ingredients:
- Pinch of cayenne pepper
- Pinch of sea salt

- Meanwhile, in a small bowl mix together the remaining ingredients.
- Drizzle the watermelon slices with the lemon mixture and serve.

63) Mango sauce

Preparation time: 15 minutes **Cooking time:** **Servings:** 6

Ingredients:
- 1 avocado, peeled, pitted and cut into cubes
- 2 tablespoons fresh lime juice
- 1 mango, peeled, pitted and cut into cubes
- 1 cup cherry tomatoes, halved

Directions:
- In a large bowl, add the avocado and lime juice and mix well.

Nutrition: Calories

Ingredients:
- 1 jalapeño bell pepper, seeded and chopped
- 1 tablespoon fresh cilantro, chopped
- Sea salt, to taste

- Add remaining ingredients and stir to combine.
- Serve immediately.

64) Avocado gazpacho

Preparation time: 15 minutes **Cooking time:** **Servings:** 6

Ingredients:
- 3 large avocados, peeled, pitted and chopped
- 1/3 cup fresh coriander leaves
- 3 cups of homemade vegetable broth
- 2 tablespoons fresh lemon juice

Directions:
- Add all ingredients to a high speed blender and pulse until smooth.

Ingredients:
- 1 teaspoon of ground cumin
- ¼ teaspoon cayenne pepper
- Sea salt, to taste

- Transfer the soup to a large bowl.
- Cover the bowl and refrigerate to chill for at least 2-3 hours before serving.

65) Roasted chickpeas

Preparation time: 10 minutes **Cooking time:** 45 minutes **Servings:** 12

Ingredients:
- ✓ 4 cups of cooked chickpeas
- ✓ 2 garlic cloves, minced
- ✓ ½ teaspoon dried oregano, crushed
- ✓ ½ teaspoon of smoked paprika

Ingredients:
- ✓ ¼ teaspoon ground cumin
- ✓ Sea salt, to taste
- ✓ 1 tablespoon of olive oil

Directions:
- ❖ Preheat oven to 400 degrees F. Grease a large baking sheet.
- ❖ Arrange the chickpeas on the prepared baking sheet in a single layer.
- ❖ Roast for about 30 minutes, stirring the chickpeas every 10 minutes.
- ❖ Meanwhile, in a small bowl, mix together garlic, thyme and spices.
- ❖ Remove the baking sheet from the oven.
- ❖ Pour the garlic mixture and oil over the chickpeas and toss to coat well.
- ❖ Roast for another 10-15 minutes or so.
- ❖ Now, turn off the oven but let the pan sit for about 10 minutes before serving.

Nutrition: Calories

66) Banana chips

Preparation time: 10 minutes **Cooking time:** 1 hour and 10 minutes **Portions:**

Ingredients:
- ✓ *2 large bananas, peeled and cut into ¼ inch thick slices*

Ingredients:

Directions:
- ❖ Prepare oven for 250 degrees F. Line a large baking sheet with baking paper.
- ❖ Arrange the banana slices on the prepared baking sheet in a single layer.
- ❖ Bake for about 1 hour.

Nutrition: Calories

67) Roasted cashews

Preparation time: 10 minutes **Cooking time:** 10 minutes **Servings:** 12

Ingredients:
- ✓ 2 cups of raw cashews
- ✓ ½ teaspoon of ground cumin
- ✓ ¼ teaspoon cayenne pepper

Ingredients:
- ✓ Pinch of salt
- ✓ 1 tablespoon fresh lemon juice

Directions:
- ❖ Preheat oven to 400 degrees F. Line a large baking sheet with a piece of foil.
- ❖ In a large bowl, add the cashews and spices and stir to coat well.
- ❖ Transfer cashews to the prepared baking dish.
- ❖ Roast for about 8-10 minutes.
- ❖ Drizzle with lemon juice and serve.

Nutrition: Calories

68) Dried orange slices

Preparation time: 10 minutes **Cooking time:** 1 hour **Servings:** 15

Ingredients:
- ✓ *4 navel oranges without seeds, cut into thin slices (DO NOT peel the oranges)*

Ingredients:

Directions:
- ❖ Set the dehydrator to 135 degrees F.
- ❖ Arrange the orange slices on the sheets of the dehydrator.
- ❖ Dehydrate for about 10 hours.

Nutrition: Calories

69) Chickpea hummus

Preparation time: 10 minutes   **Cooking time**:   **Servings**: 12

Ingredients:
- 2 (15-ounce) cans of chickpeas, rinsed and drained
- ½ cup of tahini
- 1 garlic clove, minced
- 2 tablespoons fresh lemon juice

Directions:
- In a blender, add all ingredients and pulse until smooth.

Ingredients:
- Sea salt, to taste
- Filtered water, if necessary
- 1 tablespoon olive oil plus more for spraying
- Pinch of cayenne pepper
- Transfer hummus to a large bowl and drizzle with oil.
- Sprinkle with cayenne pepper and serve immediately.

Nutrition: Calories

70) Avocado chips in the oven

Preparation time: 7 minutes   **Cooking time**: 17 minutes   **Servings**: 4

Ingredients:
- ½ cup of almond flour
- ½ teaspoon ground paprika, plus more for dusting
- 2 tablespoons of nutritional yeast
- ½ teaspoon of garlic powder

Directions:
- Preheat the oven to 420°F.
- In a small bowl, mix together the almond flour, nutritional yeast, garlic powder, paprika and salt until well combined.
- Halve and pit the avocados, and split each half from pole to pole. Remove the skin.
- Add the almond milk to another small bowl.
- Line a baking sheet with baking paper.

Ingredients:
- 2 avocados, slightly unripe
- ½ cup of almond milk
- ½ teaspoon of sea salt

- Dip an avocado slice first in the milk and then in the coating mixture, turning it gently to make sure it is completely covered, and place it on the prepared baking sheet. Repeat with the other avocado slices.
- Bake for 15-17 minutes, being careful not to overcook or burn them.
- Remove from oven, sprinkle with more paprika and serve immediately.

Nutrition: Calories

71) Dried apples with cinnamon

Preparation time: 3 minutes   **Cooking time**: 3 hours   **Servings**: 1

Ingredients:
- 2 apples, sliced
- 1 teaspoon ground cinnamon

Directions:
- Spread all the apple slices on a baking sheet.
- Cough up the slices with cinnamon and olive oil.

Ingredients:
- 1 teaspoon of olive oil

- Bake for 3 hours at 200 degrees F.
- Serve and enjoy!

Nutrition: Calories

72) Guacamole sauce

Preparation time: 5 minutes   **Cooking time**:   **Servings**: 1

Ingredients:
- ½ cup sauce,
- 2 crushed avocados,

Directions:
- Mix all ingredients together in a bowl.

Ingredients:
- 2 tablespoons of chopped coriander
- Salt, to taste

- Serve and enjoy!

Nutrition: Calories

73) Apple chip

Preparation time: 3 minutes   **Cooking time:** 40 minutes   **Servings:** 2

Ingredients:
- 2 apples, core and thin slices
- 2 tbsp white sugar

Ingredients:
- ½ teaspoon ground cinnamon

Directions:
- Preheat the oven to 225 degrees F.
- Place the apple slices on a baking sheet.
- Sprinkle with cinnamon and sugar.
- Bake for 40 minutes and then serve.

Nutrition: Calories

74) Alka-Goulash fast

Preparation time: 10 minutes   **Cooking time:** 15 minutes   **Servings:** 4

Ingredients:
- 1 onion, finely chopped
- 1 garlic clove, crushed
- 2 carrots, diced
- 3 zucchini, diced
- 2 tablespoons of olive oil
- 1 tablespoon of paprika
- ¼ teaspoon ground nutmeg

Ingredients:
- 1 tablespoon fresh parsley, chopped
- 1 tablespoon of tomato puree
- 2 cups of tomatoes, peeled
- 2 cups of cooked, drained and rinsed red beans
- ½ cup of tomato juice
- Salt and black pepper to taste

Directions:
- Sauté onion, garlic, carrot and zucchini in olive oil over medium heat for 5 minutes until softened.
- Add the paprika, nutmeg, parsley and tomato puree.
- Add the tomatoes, red beans and tomato juice and stir.
- Simmer for 10 minutes until heated through.
- Serve immediately. Enjoy!

Nutrition: Calories

75) Eggplant Caviar

Preparation time: **Cooking time:**   **Servings:** 2-4

Ingredients:
- 2 medium eggplants
- 2 tablespoons of olive oil
- 1 onion, finely chopped
- 1 green bell pepper, seedless and finely chopped
- 2 spoons of tomato puree

Ingredients:
- 4 tablespoons of water
- 2 tablespoons of lemon juice
- Salt and black pepper to taste
- Gluten-free bread or wrap of your choice

Directions:
- Pierce eggplant several times with a sharp knife. Boil or steam until soft. Allow them to cool.
- Remove stems and scoop out pulp from eggplant. Finely chop the soft pulp.
- Add the olive oil to a large skillet over medium heat. Sauté the onion and green bell pepper until the onion is translucent.
- Add the eggplant, tomato puree, water, salt and black pepper to the skillet.
- Reduce the heat and cook over low heat. Stir frequently for 20-30 minutes, at which point the mixture will begin to thicken.
- Place the mixture in a bowl and stir in the lemon juice.
- Allow the mixture to cool and place in the refrigerator.
- Serve cold with a slice of gluten-free bread, a wrap, or chopped vegetables (e.g., carrots or cucumbers).

Nutrition: Calories

76) Spiced nut mixture

Preparation time: Cooking time: Servings: 4

Ingredients:
- 1/3 cup sesame seeds
- 1/2 cup hazelnuts, blanched
- 3 tablespoons of coriander seeds
- 2 tablespoons of cumin seeds

Directions:
- Dry-fry sesame seeds in a large skillet over medium heat until golden brown. Remove from heat and let cool in a bowl.
- Toast the hazelnuts in the same pan until shiny and starting to turn golden brown. Add to the sesame seeds and let cool.
- Dry fry the coriander and cumin seeds until fragrant, but be sure not to let them burn. Add them to the bowl of nuts and sesame seeds and let cool.

Nutrition: Calories

Ingredients:
- Hot gluten-free tortillas of your choice, cut into strips or chopped vegetables
- Olive Oil
- 1/2 teaspoon salt
- Black pepper to taste

- Now place the mixture in a food processor and add salt and black pepper to taste. Process the mixture until it reaches the consistency of a coarse, dry powder.
- Serve with gluten-free tortilla wraps or veggies alongside a bowl of olive oil. To consume, dip the bread or raw veggies, into the oil and then into the spicy nut mixture.

77) Garlic mushrooms

Preparation time: Cooking time: Servings: 4

Ingredients:
- 2 tablespoons of olive oil
- 2 garlic cloves, crushed
- 1/4 teaspoon of dried thyme
- 1/4 teaspoon of dried parsley
- 1/4 teaspoon of dried sage
- 2 cups of mushrooms, cut in quarters

Directions:
- Sauté garlic in olive oil until softened and beginning to brown.
- Add the dried herbs and mushrooms and season with salt and black pepper to taste.

Nutrition: Calories

Ingredients:
- Chopped raw vegetables of your choice (e.g. cucumbers, carrots, peppers)
- 2 tablespoons chives, chopped
- Salt and black pepper to taste

- Sauté this mixture over low heat for about 10 minutes, until the mushrooms are soft.
- Serve the mushrooms alongside the raw vegetables. Garnish with the chopped chives.
- Enjoy!

78) Hummus

Preparation time: Cooking time: Portions:

Ingredients:
- 1 cup cooked chickpeas, stock reserve
- 4 tablespoons of light tahini
- Juice of 2 lemons

Directions:
- Blend chickpeas with 1/8 cup reserved broth from cooking.
- Add the lemon juice, garlic, tahini and half of the olive oil.
- Blend this mixture until smooth.

Nutrition: Calories

Ingredients:
- 6 tablespoons of olive oil
- 4 garlic cloves, crushed
- Salt to taste

- Allow to rest for about an hour before serving.
- To serve, drizzle the remaining olive oil over each individual serving. Serve alongside some raw vegetables.

79) Paleo vegan zucchini hummus

Preparation time: Cooking time: Portions:

Ingredients:
- 1 cup sliced zucchini
- 4 tablespoons of light tahini
- Juice of 2 lemons

Directions:
- Combine zucchini, lemon juice, garlic, tahini and half of the olive oil in a blender.
- Blend this mixture until smooth.

Nutrition: Calories

Ingredients:
- 6 tablespoons of olive oil
- 4 garlic cloves, crushed
- Himalayan salt to taste

- Allow to rest for about an hour before serving.
- To serve, drizzle the remaining olive oil over each individual serving. Serve alongside some raw vegetables or sprouted bread.

80) German style sweet potato salad

Preparation time: Cooking time: Servings: 2-4

Ingredients:
- 2 cups sweet potatoes, chopped
- 1 cup baby spinach
- 1 cup of cherry tomatoes
- 1 red bell pepper
- 4 tablespoons of olive oil

Directions:
- Clean and peel the potatoes. Boil them in a saucepan until tender. The time required will vary depending on their size.
- Meanwhile, sauté the garlic and scallions in a skillet over medium heat for 2-3 minutes, until slightly soft.
- Add the dill and sauté for about 1 minute.

Nutrition: Calories

Ingredients:
- 4 shallots, cut and finely chopped
- 1 garlic clove, crushed or minced
- 2 tablespoons fresh dill, finely chopped
- 2 tablespoons fresh parsley, chopped
- Salt and black pepper to taste

- Remove from heat and season to taste with salt and black pepper.
- Drain the potatoes once they are cooked, and pour the herb dressing over them while they are hot.
- Let cool and then add the rest of the ingredients and garnish with parsley. Serve fresh!

Chapter 6 - Dessert Recipes

81) Red fruit and vegetable smoothie

Preparation time: 10 minutes   Cooking time: Servings: 2

Ingredients:
- ½ cup fresh raspberries
- ½ cup fresh strawberries
- ½ red bell pepper, seeded and chopped
- ½ cup red cabbage, chopped

Directions:
- Place all ingredients in a high speed blender and pulse until creamy.

Nutrition: Calories

Ingredients:
- 1 small tomato
- 1 cup of water
- ½ cup of ice cubes

- Pour the smoothie into two glasses and serve immediately.

82) Kale Smoothie

Preparation time: 10 minutes   Cooking time: Servings: 2

Ingredients:
- 3 fresh cabbage stalks, cut and chopped
- 1-2 celery stalks, chopped
- ½ avocado, peeled, pitted and chopped

Directions:
- Place all ingredients in a high speed blender and pulse until creamy.

Nutrition: Calories

Ingredients:
- ½ inch ginger root, chopped
- ½ inch turmeric root, chopped
- 2 cups of coconut milk

- Pour the smoothie into two glasses and serve immediately.

83) Green Tofu Smoothie

Preparation time: 10 minutes   Cooking time: Servings: 2

Ingredients:
- 1½ cups cucumber, peeled and coarsely chopped
- 3 cups fresh spinach
- 2 cups of frozen broccoli
- ½ cup silken tofu, drained and pressed

Directions:
- Place all ingredients in a high speed blender and pulse until creamy.

Nutrition: Calories

Ingredients:
- 1 tablespoon fresh lime juice
- 4-5 drops of liquid stevia
- 1 cup unsweetened almond milk
- ½ cup ice, crushed
- Pour the smoothie into two glasses and serve immediately.

84) Grape and chard smoothie

Preparation time: 10 minutes   Cooking time: Servings: 2

Ingredients:
- 2 cups of green grapes without seeds
- 2 cups fresh beets, cut and chopped
- 2 tablespoons of maple syrup

Directions:
- Place all ingredients in a high speed blender and pulse until creamy.

Nutrition: Calories

Ingredients:
- 1 teaspoon fresh lemon juice
- 1½ cups of water
- 4 ice cubes

- Pour the smoothie into two glasses and serve immediately.

85) Matcha Smoothie

Preparation time: 10 minutes   **Cooking time:**   **Servings:** 2

Ingredients:
- 2 tablespoons of chia seeds
- 2 teaspoons of matcha green tea powder
- ½ teaspoon fresh lemon juice
- ½ teaspoon xanthan gum

Directions:
- Place all ingredients in a high speed blender and pulse until creamy.

Nutrition: Calories

Ingredients:
- 8-10 drops of liquid stevia
- 4 tablespoons of coconut cream
- 1½ cups unsweetened almond milk
- ¼ cup ice cubes
- Pour the smoothie into two glasses and serve immediately.

86) Banana Smoothie

Preparation time: 10 minutes   **Cooking time:**   **Servings:** 2

Ingredients:
- 2 cups of cooled unsweetened almond milk
- 1 large frozen banana, peeled and sliced

Directions:
- Place all ingredients in a high speed blender and pulse until creamy.

Nutrition: Calories

Ingredients:
- 1 tablespoon almonds, chopped
- 1 teaspoon of organic vanilla extract
- Pour the smoothie into two glasses and serve immediately.

87) Strawberry Smoothie

Preparation time: 10 minutes   **Cooking time:**   **Servings:** 2

Ingredients:
- 2 cups of cooled unsweetened almond milk
- 1½ cups of frozen strawberries

Directions:
- Add all ingredients to a high speed blender and pulse until smooth.

Nutrition: Calories

Ingredients:
- 1 banana, peeled and sliced
- ¼ teaspoon of organic vanilla extract
- Pour the smoothie into two glasses and serve immediately.

88) Raspberry and tofu smoothie

Preparation time: 15 minutes   **Cooking time:**   **Servings:** 2

Ingredients:
- 1½ cups of fresh raspberries
- 6 ounces of firm silken tofu, drained
- 1/8 teaspoon of coconut extract

Directions:
- Add all ingredients to a high speed blender and pulse until smooth.

Nutrition: Calories

Ingredients:
- 1 teaspoon of stevia powder
- 1½ cups unsweetened almond milk
- ¼ cup ice cubes, crushed
- Pour the smoothie into two glasses and serve immediately.

89) Mango Smoothie

Preparation time: 10 minutes   **Cooking time:**   **Servings:** 2

Ingredients:
- 2 cups frozen mango, peeled, pitted and chopped
- ¼ cup almond butter
- Pinch of ground turmeric

Directions:
- Add all ingredients to a high speed blender and pulse until smooth.

Nutrition: Calories

Ingredients:
- 2 tablespoons fresh lemon juice
- 1¼ cup unsweetened almond milk
- ¼ cup ice cubes

- Pour the smoothie into two glasses and serve immediately.

90) Pineapple Smoothie

Preparation time: 10 minutes   **Cooking time:**   **Servings:** 2

Ingredients:
- 2 cups pineapple, chopped
- ½ teaspoon fresh ginger, peeled and chopped
- ½ teaspoon ground turmeric
- 1 teaspoon of natural immune support supplement*.

Directions:
- Add all ingredients to a high speed blender and pulse until smooth.

Nutrition: Calories

Ingredients:
- 1 teaspoon of chia seeds
- 1½ cups of cold green tea
- ½ cup ice, crushed

- Pour the smoothie into two glasses and serve immediately.

91) Cabbage and pineapple smoothie

Preparation time: 15 minutes   **Cooking time:**   **Servings:** 2

Ingredients:
- 1½ cups fresh cabbage, chopped and shredded
- 1 frozen banana, peeled and chopped
- ½ cup of fresh pineapple chunks

Directions:
- Add all ingredients to a high speed blender and pulse until smooth.

Nutrition: Calories

Ingredients:
- 1 cup unsweetened coconut milk
- ½ cup of fresh orange juice
- ½ cup of ice

- Pour the smoothie into two glasses and serve immediately.

92) Green Vegetable Smoothie

Preparation time: 15 minutes   **Cooking time:**   **Servings:** 2

Ingredients:
- 1 medium avocado, peeled, pitted and chopped
- 1 large cucumber, peeled and chopped
- 2 fresh tomatoes, chopped
- 1 small green bell pepper, seeded and chopped

Directions:
- Add all ingredients to a high speed blender and pulse until smooth.

Nutrition: Calories

Ingredients:
- 1 cup fresh spinach, torn
- 2 tablespoons fresh lime juice
- 2 tablespoons of homemade vegetable broth
- 1 cup of alkaline water
- Pour smoothie into glasses and serve immediately.

93) Avocado and spinach smoothie

Preparation time: 10 minutes   **Cooking time:**   **Servings:** 2

Ingredients:
- 2 cups of fresh spinach
- ½ avocado, peeled, pitted and chopped
- 4-6 drops of liquid stevia

Ingredients:
- ½ teaspoon ground cinnamon
- 1 tablespoon of hemp seeds
- 2 cups of cooled alkaline water

Directions:
- Add all ingredients to a high speed blender and pulse until smooth.
- Pour the smoothie into two glasses and serve immediately.

Nutrition: Calories

94) Cucumber Smoothie

Preparation time: 15 minutes   **Cooking time:**   **Servings:** 2

Ingredients:
- 1 small cucumber, peeled and chopped
- 2 cups fresh mixed greens (spinach, kale, chard), chopped and shredded
- ½ cup of lettuce, torn
- ¼ cup fresh parsley leaves
- ¼ cup fresh mint leaves

Ingredients:
- 2-3 drops of liquid stevia
- 1 teaspoon fresh lemon juice
- 1½ cups of filtered water
- ¼ cup ice cubes

Directions:
- Add all ingredients to a high speed blender and pulse until smooth.
- Pour the smoothie into two glasses and serve immediately.

Nutrition: Calories

95) Apple and Ginger Smoothie

Preparation time: 10 minutes   **Cooking time:** 0 minutes   **Servings:** 1

Ingredients:
- 1 apple, peeled and diced
- ¾ cup (6 ounces) of coconut yogurt

Ingredients:
- ½ teaspoon of ginger, freshly grated

Directions:
- Add all ingredients to a blender.
- Blend well until smooth.
- Refrigerate for 2 to 3 hours.
- Serve.

Nutrition: Calories

96) Green Tea Blueberry Smoothie

Preparation time: 10 minutes   **Cooking time:** 5 minutes   **Servings:** 1

Ingredients:
- 3 tablespoons of alkaline water
- 1 green tea bag
- 1 ½ cups fresh blueberries

Ingredients:
- 1 pear, peeled, stoned and diced
- ¾ cup of almond milk

Directions:
- Boil 3 tablespoons of water in a small saucepan and transfer to a cup.
- Dip the tea bag into the cup and let it sit for 4 to 5 minutes.
- Discard the tea bag and
- Transfer the green tea to a blender
- Add all other ingredients to blender.
- Blend well until smooth.
- Serve with fresh blueberries.

Nutrition: Calories

97) Apple and almond smoothie

Preparation time: 10 minutes **Cooking time:** 0 minutes **Servings:** 1

Ingredients:
- 1 cup of apple cider
- 1/2 cup of coconut yogurt
- 4 tablespoons almonds, crushed

Directions:
- Add all ingredients to a blender.

Ingredients:
- 1/4 teaspoon of cinnamon
- 1/4 teaspoon nutmeg
- 1 cup of ice cubes
- Blend well until smooth.
- Serve.

Nutrition: Calories

98) Cranberry Smoothie

Preparation time: 10 minutes **Cooking time:** 0 minutes **Servings:** 1

Ingredients:
- 1 cup of cranberries
- ¾ cup of almond milk
- ¼ cup raspberries

Directions:
- Add all ingredients to a blender.

Ingredients:
- 2 teaspoons fresh ginger, finely grated
- 2 teaspoons of fresh lemon juice
- Blend well until smooth.
- Serve with fresh berries on top.

Nutrition: Calories

99) Berry and Cinnamon Smoothie

Preparation time: 10 minutes **Cooking time:** 0 minutes **Servings:** 1

Ingredients:
- 1 cup of frozen strawberries
- 1 cup apple, peeled and diced
- 2 teaspoons fresh ginger
- 3 tablespoons of hemp seeds

Directions:
- Add all ingredients to a blender.

Ingredients:
- 1 cup of water
- ½ squeezed lime
- ¼ teaspoon of cinnamon powder
- ⅛ teaspoon of vanilla extract
- Blend well until smooth.
- Serve with fresh fruit

Nutrition: Calories

100) Detoxifying Berry Smoothie

Preparation time: 10 minutes **Cooking time:** 0 minutes **Servings:** 1

Ingredients:
- 3 peaches, with stone and peel
- 5 blueberries

Directions:
- Add all ingredients to a blender.

Ingredients:
- 5 raspberries
- 1 cup of alkaline water
- Blend well until smooth.
- Serve with fresh kiwi wedges.

Nutrition: Calories

Chapter 7 - Dr. Lewis's Meal Plan Project

Day 1

1) Bowl Of Raspberry And Banana Smoothie
21) Tomato And Vegetable Salad
43) Spaghetti With Broccoli
62) Grilled Watermelon
85) Matcha Smoothie

Day 2

5) Spicy Quinoa Porridge
25) Curried Okra
48) Fresh Vegetarian Pizza
68) Dried Orange Slices
82) Kale Smoothie

Day 3

8) Fruity Oatmeal
28) Sauteed Mushrooms
56) Mint And Berry Soup
65) Roasted Chickpeas
94) Cucumber Smoothie

Day 4

11) Savory Sweet Potato Waffles
31) Roasted Butternut Squash
59) Mixed Mushroom Stew
74) Alka-Goulash Fast
91) Cabbage And Pineapple Smoothie

Day 5

14) Simple White Bread
34) Vegetarian Kebab
49) Spicy Lentil Burger
80) German Style Sweet Potato Salad
89) Mango Smoothie

Day 6

17) Granola With Coconut, Nuts And Seeds
37) Zoodles With Cream Sauce
57) Mushroom Soup
75) Eggplant Caviar
96) Green Tea Blueberry Smoothie

Day 7

20) Strawberry Sorbet
40) Vegetable Dish With Sesame
51) Sliced Sweet Potato With Artichoke Cream And Peppers
78) Hummus
99) Berry And Cinnamon Smoothie

Chapter 8 - Conclusion

I hope this book can lead you to your goals, keeping your desire to keep going high, without making you lose sight of the outcome

This book series is designed to help women, men, athletes and sportsmen, people immersed in work with little free time, etc.

If you recognize yourself in one of these categories or someone you know has decided to take the same path as you,

You'll find the other books in the series in your trusted bookstore, guaranteed!

Big hugs from Dr. Grace!

Alkaline Diet Cookbook for Men

Dr. Lewis's Meal Plan Project| 100 Specific Recipes to Keep Body Acids Under Control| Find the Well-Being You've Always Wished For Thanks to an Effective and Easy-To-Follow Path.

By Grace Lewis

Chapter 1 - Introduction

This book was written for all men who have made the choice to embark on a journey of transforming their lives.

The alkaline diet is the simplest and most effective way to begin a long-term journey of transformation.

Below we will answer some questions that people usually ask me during private sessions

What is an alkaline diet?

The premise of an alkaline diet is this: replace acidic foods with alkaline foods and your health will improve. Why would this work, you may ask? The theory is that by regulating your body's pH level (pH is a scientific scale on which acids and bases are measured), you can lose weight and avoid chronic diseases such as cancer and heart disease. pH is measured on a scale of 1 to 14; below seven are the most acidic foods, such as vinegar, animal fats and dairy products. Above seven are the alkaline foods, which mostly include healthy, plant-based foods. When we digest a food, we are left with residual ash, which can be acidic or alkaline. Therefore, an alkaline diet is sometimes called an alkaline ash diet. Proponents of the alkaline diet say that acidic ash can be dangerous to your health.

Is an alkaline diet healthy?

Processed meats are high on cancer doctors' list of foods never to eat, and they are also condemned in the alkaline diet because of their high acidity. "An alkaline diet is a diet that seeks to balance the body's pH levels by increasing the consumption of alkalizing foods such as fruits and vegetables and reducing/eliminating most acidifying foods such as processed meats and refined grains," explains Josh Axe, DNM, author of Eat Dirt and co-founder of Ancient Nutrition.

Can an alkaline diet reduce the risk of cancer?

Many anti-cancer foods are also alkaline diet foods, but there is currently no evidence for or against the role of alkaline diets in cancer prevention. However, plant-based diets are thought to help reduce the risk of cancer and are even recommended for cancer survivors, according to the American Institute for Cancer Research. New research from the University of Alabama at Birmingham suggests that a plant-based diet may make it easier to treat one of the deadliest forms of breast cancer. Although the evidence is somewhat contradictory: some chemotherapy drugs kill more cancer cells in an alkaline environment, while others work better in an acidic environment, according to a review in the Journal of Environmental Public Health. It's worth discussing this with your doctor if you are being treated for cancer.

At the end of the manual, you'll find my personal method designed for a male audience to get you started on the recipes in this book right away.

Enjoy!

Grace

Chapter 2 - Breakfast Recipes

1) *Blueberry Muffins*

Preparation time: 1 hour **Cooking time:** **Servings:** 3

Ingredients:
- ✓ 1/2 cup of Blueberries
- ✓ 3/4 cup of Teff Flour
- ✓ 3/4 cup of Spelt Flour
- ✓ 1/3 cup of Agave Syrup

Ingredients:
- ✓ 1/2 teaspoon of Pure Sea Salt
- ✓ 1 cup of Coconut Milk
- ✓ 1/4 cup Sea Moss Gel seed oil (optional, check information)

Directions:
- ❖ Preheat our oven to 365 degrees Fahrenheit.
- ❖ Grate or line up 6 standard muffin cups.
- ❖ Add the yeast, sifted flour, sifted mashed potato, nut milk, peanut butter, and agave juice to a large bowl.
- ❖ Put them in order for a while.
- ❖ Add the blueberries to the mixture and mix well.
- ❖ Divide muffin batter among 6 muffin cups.
- ❖ Bake for 30 minutes until golden brown.
- ❖ Experiment and enjoy our Blueberry Muffins!

Nutrition: Calories

Helpful Hints:

2) *Banana Strawberry Ice Crem*

Preparation time: **Cooking time:** 4 Hours **Servings:** 5

Ingredients:
- ✓ 1 cup of Strawberry*.
- ✓ 5 quartered Baby Bananas*.
- ✓ 1/2 Avocado, chopped

Ingredients:
- ✓ 1 tablespoon of Agave syrup
- ✓ 1/4 cup of walnut milk Homemade

Directions:
- ❖ Put all the ingredients in and let them dry well.
- ❖ Taste. If so, add more milk or agave syrup if you want it to be more full-bodied.
- ❖ Place in a container with a lid and let mash for at least 5-6 hours.
- ❖ Serve and enjoy your Bana Strawberry Ice creamy!

Nutrition: Calories

Helpful hints: If you don't fresh berries or banas, you can use frozen ones. You can use as much fruit as you want, but be sure to use only fresh fruit. The fat in the Avocado helps make a creamier consistency. If you don't have homemade nut milk, you can substitute it with homemade sheep's milk.

3) *Chocolate cream Homemade Whipped*

Preparation time: 10 Minutes.   **Cooking time:**   **Servings:** 1 cup

Ingredients:
- 1 cup of Aquafaba

Directions:
- Add Agave Syrup and Aquafaba into a bowl.
- Mix to the height speed about 5 minutes with a mixer stand o 10 to 15 minutes with a mixer hand.

Nutrition: Calories

Ingredients:
- 1/4 cup of Agave Syrup
- Serve and enjoy our Homemade Whipped Cream!

Helpful Hints: Keep in the refrigerator if not using immediately. The whipped cream will become Aquafaba consistency eventually, until set.

4) *"Chocolate" Pudding.*

Preparation time: **Cooking time:** 20 Minutes.   **Servings:** 4

Ingredients:
- 1 to 2 cups of Black Sapote
- 1/4 cup agave syrup
- 1/2 cup of soaked Brazil Nuts (overnight or at least 3 hours)

Directions:
- Cut 1 or 2 cups of Black Sapote in half.
- Remove all the seeds. You should have 1 cup ou full of fruit de-seded.

Nutrition: Calories

Ingredients:
- 1 tablespoon of hemp seeds
- 1/2 cup of Spring Water
- Place all ingredients in a blender and blend until smooth.
- Serve and enjoy our chocolate pudding!

Helpful Hints: Store in the refrigerator when not in use. You can use it with our Homemade whipped crust.

5) *Walnut muffins*

Preparation time: **Cooking time:** 1 hour   **Servings:** 6

Ingredients:
- Dry ingredients:
- 1 1/2 cups of Spell or Teff Flour
- 1/2 teaspoon of Pure Sea Salt
- 3/4 cup of Date Syrup
- What's the problem?
- 2 medium pureed Burro Banas

Directions:
- Preheat the oven to 400 degrees.
- Take a muffin tray and grease 12 cups or line with cupcake liners.
- Place all dry ingredients in a large bowl and mix well.
- Add all ingredients to a larger bowl and mix with the Bin Laden. 5. Mix the ingredients from the two bowls into one container. Be careful not to over mix.

Nutrition: Calories

Ingredients:
- ¼ cup of ground soybean oil
- ¾ cup of Homemade Walnut Milk *
- 1 tablespoon of Key Lime Juice
- Ingredients for filling:
- ½ cup of chopped Walnuts (plus extra for decorating)
- 1 banana burrita
- Add the filling ingredients and fry.
- Place our batter in the 12 muffin cups and fill them with a knob of butter.
- Bake 22 to 26 mnutes until golden brown.
- Allow to cool for 10 minutes.
- Serve and enjoy your Bana Nut Muffins!

Helpful Hints:

6) *Banana and almond smoothie*

Preparation time: 10 minutes   **Cooking time:** 0 minutes   **Servings:** 2

Ingredients:
- 2 large frozen bananas, peeled and sliced
- 1 tablespoon chopped almonds

Directions:
- ❖ Place all ingredients in a high speed blender and pulse until smooth and creamy.

Nutrition: Calories

Ingredients:
- 1 teaspoon of organic vanilla extract
- 2 cups of cooled unsweetened almond milk

- ❖ Pour smoothie into two serving glasses and serve immediately

7) *Strawberry and Beet Smoothie*

Preparation time: 10 minutes   **Cooking time:** 0 minutes   **Servings:** 2

Ingredients:
- 2 cups frozen strawberries, hulled
- 2/3 cup frozen beets, cut, peeled and chopped
- 1 teaspoon of fresh ginger root, peeled and grated

Directions:
- ❖ Place all ingredients in a high speed blender and pulse until smooth and creamy.

Nutrition: Calories

Ingredients:
- 1 teaspoon fresh turmeric root, peeled and grated
- ½ cup of fresh orange juice
- 1 cup unsweetened almond milk

- ❖ Pour smoothie into two serving glasses and serve immediately

8) *Raspberry and tofu smoothie*

Preparation time: 10 minutes   **Cooking time:**   **Servings:** 2

Ingredients:
- 1½ cups of fresh raspberries
- 6 ounces of firm silken tofu, drained, pressed and chopped
- 1 teaspoon of stevia powder

Directions:
- ❖ Place all ingredients in a high speed blender and pulse until smooth and creamy.

Nutrition: Calories

Ingredients:
- 1/8 teaspoon of organic vanilla extract
- 1½ cups unsweetened almond milk
- ¼ cup ice cubes, crushed

- ❖ Pour smoothie into two serving glasses and serve immediately

9) *Mango and lemon smoothie*

Preparation time: 10 minutes   **Cooking time:**   **Servings:** 2

Ingredients:
- 2 cups frozen mango, peeled, pitted and chopped
- ¼ cup almond butter
- pinch of ground turmeric

Directions:
- ❖ Place all ingredients in a high speed blender and pulse until smooth and creamy.

Nutrition: Calories

Ingredients:
- 2 tablespoons fresh lemon juice
- 1¼ cup unsweetened almond milk
- ¼ cup ice cubes, crushed

- ❖ Pour smoothie into two serving glasses and serve immediately

10) Papaya and banana smoothie

Preparation time: 10 minutes   **Cooking time**:   **Servings**: 2

Ingredients:
- ½ of a medium papaya, peeled and coarsely chopped
- 1 large banana, peeled and sliced
- 2 tablespoons of agave nectar
- ¼ teaspoon ground turmeric

Directions:
- Place all ingredients in a high speed blender and pulse until smooth and creamy.

Nutrition: Calories

Ingredients:
- 1 tablespoon fresh lime juice
- 1½ cups unsweetened almond milk
- ½ cup ice cubes, crushed

- Pour smoothie into two serving glasses and serve immediately

11) Orange and Oat Smoothie

Preparation time: 10 minutes   **Cooking time**:   **Servings**: 2

Ingredients:
- 2/3 cups rolled oats
- 2 oranges, peeled, with seeds and cut into pieces
- 2 large bananas, peeled and sliced

Directions:
- Place all ingredients in a high speed blender and pulse until smooth and creamy.

Nutrition: Calories

Ingredients:
- 1½ cups unsweetened almond milk
- ½ cup ice cubes, crushed

- Pour smoothie into two serving glasses and serve immediately

12) Pineapple and Kale Smoothie

Preparation time: 10 minutes   **Cooking time**:   **Servings**: 2

Ingredients:
- 1½ cups fresh cabbage, hard ribs removed and chopped
- 1 large frozen banana, peeled and sliced
- ½ cup fresh pineapple, peeled and cut into pieces

Directions:
- Place all ingredients in a high speed blender and pulse until smooth and creamy.

Nutrition: Calories

Ingredients:
- ½ cup of fresh orange juice
- 1 cup unsweetened coconut milk
- ½ cup ice cubes, crushed

- Pour smoothie into two serving glasses and serve immediately

13) Pumpkin and Banana Smoothie

Preparation time: 10 minutes   **Cooking time**:   **Servings**: 2

Ingredients:
- 1 cup homemade pumpkin puree
- 1 large banana, peeled and sliced
- 1 tablespoon maple syrup
- 1 teaspoon ground flax seeds

Directions:
- Place all ingredients in a high speed blender and pulse until smooth and creamy.

Nutrition: Calories

Ingredients:
- ¼ teaspoon of cinnamon powder
- 1/8 teaspoon ground ginger
- 1½ cups unsweetened almond milk
- ¼ cup ice cubes, crushed

- Pour smoothie into two serving glasses and serve immediately

14) Cabbage and avocado smoothie

Preparation time: 10 minutes   **Cooking time**:   **Servings**: 2

Ingredients:
- 2 cups fresh cabbage, hard ribs removed and chopped
- ½ of a medium avocado, peeled, pitted and chopped
- ½ inch pieces of fresh ginger root, peeled and chopped

Directions:
- Place all ingredients in a high speed blender and pulse until smooth and creamy.

Nutrition: Calories

Ingredients:
- ½ inch pieces of fresh turmeric root, peeled and chopped
- 1½ cups unsweetened coconut milk
- ¼ cup ice cubes, crushed
- Pour smoothie into two serving glasses and serve immediately

15) Cucumber and Herb Smoothie

Preparation time: 10 minutes   **Cooking time**:   **Servings**: 2

Ingredients:
- 2 cups fresh mixed vegetables (cabbage, beets), chopped and shredded
- 1 small cucumber, peeled and chopped
- ½ cup of lettuce, torn
- ¼ cup fresh parsley leaves
- ¼ cup fresh mint leaves

Directions:
- Place all ingredients in a high speed blender and pulse until smooth and creamy.

Nutrition: Calories

Ingredients:
- 2-3 drops of liquid stevia
- 1 teaspoon fresh lemon juice
- 1½ cups of alkaline water
- ¼ cup ice cubes, crushed

16) Hemp seed and carrot muffins

Pour smoothie into two serving glasses and serve immediately

Preparation time: 20-25 minutes   **Cooking time**:   **Servings**: 12

Ingredients:
- Cashew butter, 6 tablespoons
- Shredded Carrot,
- Unrefined whole cane sugar, .5 c.
- Almond milk, 1 c.
- Oatmeal, 2 c.
- Ground flaxseed, 1 tablespoon

Directions:
- Start by setting your oven to 350.
- Whisk the flax seeds and water together to make the flax egg.
- Pour everything into a larger bowl and then combine the salt, vanilla powder, baking powder, kale, hemp seeds, cashew butter, carrot, sugar, almond milk and oatmeal.

Nutrition: Calories

Ingredients:
- Water, 3 tablespoons
- Pinch of sea salt
- Powdered vanilla bean, one pinch
- Baking powder, 1 tablespoon
- Chopped cabbage, 1 tablespoon
- Hemp seeds, 2 tablespoons
- Mix everything together until well combined.
- Grease a 12-cup muffin pan and divide the batter between the cups. Bake for 20-25 minutes and enjoy.

17) Chia seed and strawberry parfait

Preparation time: **Cooking time:** **Servings: 2**

Ingredients:
- Strawberry mixture -
- Brown rice syrup, 1-2 teaspoons
- Chia seeds, 1 teaspoon
- Diced strawberries, 1 c.
- Oat Blend -

Directions:
- To make the strawberry mixture, mix together the brown rice syrup, chia seeds and strawberries in a small bowl until well blended.
- In a separate bowl, mix together the vanilla bean powder, brown rice syrup, coconut milk and oats until well blended.

Nutrition: Calories

Ingredients:
- Quick rolled oats, 1 c.
- Powdered vanilla bean, one pinch
- Brown rice syrup, 1 tablespoon
- Coconut milk, 1 c.

- Place one part of the oats in the base of two jars. Cover with some of the strawberry mixture. Repeat with the remaining ingredients.
- Put a lid on the jars and let them sit in the fridge overnight.
- The next morning, discover and enjoy.

18) Pecan Pancakes

Preparation time: **Cooking time:** **Servings: 5**

Ingredients:
- Chopped pecans, .25 c.
- Nutmeg, .25 tsp
- Cinnamon, 0.5 teaspoons
- Vanilla, 1 teaspoon
- Melted butter, 2 tablespoons
- Unsweetened soy milk, .75 c.

Directions:
- Place the salt, sugar substitute, baking powder and almond flour in a bowl and mix well.
- In another bowl, place the vanilla, soy milk, butter and eggs. Stir well to incorporate everything.
- Place the egg mixture into the dry contents and mix well until well blended.
- Add the nutmeg, pecans and cinnamon. Stir for five minutes.

Nutrition: Calories

Ingredients:
- Eggs, 2
- Salt, .25 tsp
- Baking powder, .25 tsp
- Granular sugar substitute, 1 tablespoon
- Almond flour, .75 c.
- Olive oil - cooking spray

- Place a 12-inch skillet over medium heat and sprinkle with cooking spray.
- Pour one tablespoon of batter into the preheated pan and spread into a four-inch circle.
- Pour three more spoonfuls into the pan and cook until bubbles have formed at the edges of the pancakes and the bottom is golden brown.
- Turn each one over and cook an additional two minutes.
- Repeat the process until all the batter has been used.
- Serve with a syrup of your choice.

19) Quinoa Breakfast

Preparation time: **Cooking time:** **Servings: 4**

Ingredients:
- Maple syrup, 3 tablespoons
- 2 inch cinnamon stick
- Water, 2 c.
- Quinoa, 1 c.
- Optional Condiments:
- Yogurt
- Chopped cashews, 2 tablespoons

Directions:
- Place the quinoa in a colander and rinse under cold running water. Make sure there are no stones or anything else.
- Pour the water into a saucepan, add the quinoa and place the saucepan over medium heat. Bring to a boil.

Nutrition: Calories

Ingredients:
- Whipped coconut cream, 3 tablespoons
- Lime juice, 1 teaspoon
- Nutmeg, .25 tsp
- Raisins, 2 tablespoons
- Strawberries, .5 c.
- Raspberries, .5 c.
- Blueberries, .5 c.

- Add the cinnamon stick, put a lid on the saucepan, lower the hot temperature, even, simmer gently fifteen minutes until the water is engulfed.
- Remove from hot temperature and stir with a fork. Add maple syrup and one of the toppings listed above.

20) Oatmeal

Preparation time: **Cooking time:** **Servings: 4**

Ingredients:
- ✓ Halls
- ✓ Steel cut oats, 1.25 c.
- ✓ Water, 3.75 c.
- ✓ Optional Condiments:
- ✓ Nuts
- ✓ Dried fruits
- ✓ Sliced banana
- ✓ Mango cubes

Ingredients:
- ✓ Mixed berries
- ✓ Garam masala, 1 teaspoon
- ✓ Lemon pepper, .25 tsp
- ✓ Nutmeg, .25 tsp
- ✓ Cinnamon, 1 teaspoon

Directions:
- ❖ Place a saucepan on medium and add the water. Allow the water to boil.
- ❖ Pour in the oats with a pinch of salt and lower the heat to a simmer.
- ❖ Let simmer 25 minutes, stirring constantly.
- ❖ Once all the water has been absorbed, add one of the seasonings listed above if you want to add some flavor. If you want it creamier, add a tablespoon of coconut milk.

Nutrition: Calories

Chapter 3 - Lunch Recipes

21) Sweet spinach salad

Preparation time: **Cooking time:**   **Portions:**

Ingredients:
- Crushed black pepper (1 teaspoon)
- Salt (1 teaspoon)
- Nutmeg (1 teaspoon)
- Cinnamon (1 teaspoon)
- Chopped spinach (4 c.)
- Chopped parsley (2 tablespoons)

Ingredients:
- Chopped walnuts (.25 c.)
- Raisins (.25 c.)
- Sliced apple (.5 c.)
- Yogurt (.5 c.)
- Lime juice (1 tablespoon)
- Shredded carrots (.75 c.)

Directions:
- To start this recipe, bring out a large bowl and combine all the ingredients together.
- Place the bowl in the refrigerator to chill for about ten minutes before serving.

Nutrition: Calories

22) Steamed green bowl

Preparation time: **Cooking time:**   **Portions:**

Ingredients:
- Chopped coriander (2 tablespoons)
- Salt (1 teaspoon)
- Sliced green onions (2)
- Ground cashews (1 c.)
- Coconut milk (2 c.)
- Green peas (.5 c.)
- Sliced zucchini (1)

Ingredients:
- Head of broccoli (1)
- Grated ginger (1 inch)
- Turmeric (1 teaspoon)
- Chopped garlic clove (1)
- Sliced onion (1)
- Coconut oil (1 tablespoon)

Directions:
- Heat some coconut oil in a pan and when hot, add the ginger, turmeric, garlic and onion.
- After five minutes of cooking, add the coconut milk, peas, zucchini and broccoli to this mixture.
- Let the ingredients come to a boil before reducing the heat and simmering for a bit.
- After another 15 minutes, stir in the cilantro, salt, green onions and cashews before serving.

Nutrition: Calories

23) Vegetable and berry salad

Preparation time: **Cooking time:**   **Portions:**

Ingredients:
- Raspberries (.5 c.)
- Sliced tangerine (.5)
- Alfalfa sprouts (1 c.)
- Shredded red cabbage (.5 head)
- Lemon juice 1
- Olive oil (3 tablespoons)
- Diced cucumber (1)
- Avocado (1)
- Sliced shallot (1)

Ingredients:
- Sliced cabbage (4 leaves)
- Chopped parsley (1 tablespoon)
- Sliced red bell pepper (.5)
- Shredded Carrot (1)
- Crushed almonds (1 tablespoon)
- Pumpkin seeds (2 tablespoons)

Directions:
- Take a large bowl and add all the ingredients to it.
- Stir well to combine before seasoning the fruits and vegetables with a little lemon juice and a little oil.
- Serve immediately.

Nutrition: Calories

24) Bowl of quinoa and carrots

Preparation time: **Cooking time:**   **Portions:**

Ingredients:
- Sliced green onions (2 tablespoons)
- Black sesame seeds (2 tablespoons)
- Salt (.25 tsp.)
- Chopped parsley (3 tablespoons)
- Lemon juice (.5)
- Cooked quinoa (2 c.)

Ingredients:
- Sliced fennel bulb (1)
- Carrots, chopped (1 bunch)
- Olive oil (1 tablespoon)
- Miso (1 tablespoon)
- Water (1 c.)

Directions:
- Whisk together the miso and water in a bowl. Then take a frying pan and heat some oil in it.
- When the oil is hot, add the fennel bulb and carrots and cook for a few minutes, turning when three minutes have passed.
- Add the water and miso mixture to the pan and reduce the heat to low. Cook with the lid on for a bit. This will take about 20 minutes.
- While this mixture is cooking, combine together the quinoa with the parsley, lemon juice and salt in a bowl.
- When the carrots are done, add the mixture on top of the quinoa. Sprinkle the green onions and sesame seeds on top before serving.

Nutrition: Calories

25) Grab and Go Wraps

Preparation time: **Cooking time:**   **Portions:**

Ingredients:
- Carrot cut into julienne (1)
- Red bell pepper (.5)
- Swiss chard greens (4)
- Salt (.25 tsp.)
- Diced jalapeno bell pepper (.5)

Ingredients:
- Shallots cut into small cubes (1)
- Chopped coriander leaves (.25 c.)
- Lime Juice (1)
- Avocado (1)
- Steamed green peas (1 c.)

Directions:
- Get out your blender or food processor and combine together the salt, jalapeno, shallots, cilantro, lime, avocado and peas. Process to combine, but leave some texture to still be there.
- Lay the collards out on the counter and then spread your pea and avocado mixture on top.
- Add the carrot and bell bell pepper strips before rolling up the collars and secure with a toothpick.
- Repeat with all ingredients before serving.

Nutrition: Calories

26) Walnut Tacos

Preparation time: **Cooking time:**   **Portions:**

Ingredients:
- Chopped coriander (1 tablespoon)
- Nutritional yeast (2 tablespoons)
- Romaine lettuce leaves (6)
- Cooked red quinoa (.25 c.)
- Salt (.25 tsp.)
- Tamari (1 tablespoon)
- Coconut amino acids (1 teaspoon)
- Smoked paprika (.25 tsp.)

Ingredients:
- Onion powder (.25 tsp.)
- Garlic Powder (.25 tsp.)
- Chilli powder (.25 tsp.)
- Ground Coriander (1 teaspoon)
- Ground Cumin (1 teaspoon)
- Olive oil (2 tablespoons)
- Chopped dried tomatoes (.25 c.)
- Chopped raw almonds (.25 c.)
- Walnuts (.5 c.)

Directions:
- To start this recipe, add the almonds and walnuts to the food processor and puree them.
- Add the tomatoes and give it a couple of pulses until you have a nice crumbly mixture.
- From there, add the salt, tamari, coconut aminos, paprika, onion, garlic, chili, cilantro, cumin, and olive oil.
- It pulses a few more times to be fully combined.
- Add the tomato and walnut mixture to a bowl and combine with the quinoa.
- Divide this mixture among the romaine lettuce leaves and top with the cilantro and nutritional yeast before serving.

Nutrition: Calories

27) Tex-Mex bowl

Preparation time: **Cooking time:** **Portions:**

Ingredients:
- Nutritional yeast (2 tablespoons)
- Cilantro (2 tablespoons)
- Sliced avocado (1)
- Salt (.25 tsp.)
- Olive oil (.25 c.)
- Apple Cider Vinegar (.25 c.)
- Lime juice and zest (1)
- Lemon juice and zest (1)
- Squeezed Oranges (2)
- Chopped garlic cloves (2)
- Sliced red onion (1)
- Sliced peppers
- For the brown rice
- Hind beans (.5 c.)

Directions:
- Pull out a large bowl and combine together the salt, olive oil, vinegar, lime zest and juice, lemon zest and juice, garlic, red onion, and bell bell pepper.
- Cover and let sit for about five hours to marinate a bit. While the peppers marinate a bit in the refrigerator, it's time to work on the sauce.
- To make the sauce, add all ingredients to a small bowl and mix well to combine. Cover the bowl and place in the refrigerator.

Nutrition: Calories

Ingredients:
- Garlic powder (.5 tsp.)
- Cayenne pepper (.5 tsp.)
- Paprika (1 teaspoon)
- Salt (1 teaspoon)
- Garlic powder (1.5 teaspoons)
- Chili powder (2 teaspoons)
- Cooked brown rice (1 c.)
- Sauce
- Juice of a lime
- Salt (.25 tsp.)
- Diced Cilantro (.25 c.)
- Diced red onion (.5)
- Diced Tomatoes (2)

- In a medium bowl, add all the ingredients for the brown rice. Mix well and set aside.
- Heat your skillet and add the peppers with some of the marinade. Cook for a bit until the onion and peppers are soft.
- Add the rice to a few serving bowls and top with the bell pepper and onion mixture, salsa and avocado. Add the nutritional yeast and cilantro before serving.

28) Avocado and salmon soup

Preparation time: **Cooking time:** **Portions:**

Ingredients:
- Cilantro (2 tablespoons)
- Crushed pepper (1 teaspoon)
- Olive oil (1 tablespoon)
- Flaked salmon (1 can)
- Salt (.25 tsp.)
- Cumin (.25 tsp.)
- Vegetable stock (1.5 c.)

Directions:
- Take out a blender and combine together the salt, cumin, vegetable broth, coconut cream, two tablespoons of lemon juice, green onion, scallion, and avocado.
- Blend until smooth and then chill in the refrigerator for an hour.

Nutrition: Calories

Ingredients:
- Whole coconut cream (2 tablespoons)
- Lemon juice (4 tablespoons)
- Sliced green onion (1 tablespoon)
- Chopped Shallot (1)
- Pitted Avocado (3)

- Meanwhile, take a bowl and combine together a tablespoon of cilantro, two tablespoons of lemon juice, the pepper, olive oil and salmon.
- Add the cooled avocado soup to the bowls and top each with the salmon and the rest of the cilantro. Serve immediately.

29) Asian Pumpkin Salad

Preparation time: **Cooking time:**   **Portions:**

Ingredients:
- Diced avocado (.5)
- Pomegranate seeds (.25 c.)
- Lemon juice (1 tablespoon)
- Sliced cabbage (4 c.)
- Olive oil (1.5 tablespoons)
- Diced pumpkin (2 c.)
- Salt (.5 tsp.)
- Red pepper flakes (.25 tsp.)
- Ground mustard (.25 tsp.)
- Ground Garlic (.25 tsp.)
- Ground cloves (.25 tsp.)
- Black sesame seeds (1 tablespoon)
- White sesame seeds (1 tablespoon)

Directions:
- Turn on the oven and give it time to heat to 400 degrees. Prepare a baking sheet with baking paper.
- In a large dish, combine the black and white sesame seeds with the salt, chili flakes, mustard, garlic and cloves.
- Drizzle the squash with a little olive oil and then roll each cube in the sesame seed mixture, pressing down a little to coat it.
- Add the squash to the baking dish and place it in the oven. It will take about half an hour to bake.
- While the squash is cooking, add the kale to a large bowl and pour in the salt, lemon juice and the rest of the olive oil. Massage the mixture into the kale and then set aside.
- When the squash is ready, add it on top of the kale and garnish with the avocado and pomegranate seeds before serving.

Nutrition: Calories

30) Sweet potato rolls

Preparation time: **Cooking time:**   **Portions:**

Ingredients:
- Avocado (1)
- Alfalfa sprouts (1 c.)
- Sliced red onion (.5)
- Spinach (1 c.)
- Cooked quinoa (.5 c.)
- Swiss chard greens (4)
- Sweet potato hummus
- Crushed black pepper (.25 tsp.)
- Salt (.25 tsp.)
- Cinnamon powder (.25 tsp.)
- Chilli powder (.25 tsp.)
- Garlic clove (1)
- Lemon juice (.5)
- Olive oil (.25 c.)
- Tahini (.33 c.)
- Diced sweet potato (1)

Directions:
- Take the sweet potatoes and add them to a pan. Cover with water and bring to a boil. When it reaches a boil, reduce the flame and let it cook for a while to make the potatoes tender.
- When these are ready, drain the water and add them to the food processor along with pepper, salt, cinnamon, chili powder, garlic, lemon juice, olive oil and tahini.
- Process until the mixture is smooth.
- Lay out each of the green collars and then spread sweet potato hummus on each.
- Add the avocado, sprouts, onion, spinach and quinoa. Roll everything up and secure with toothpicks. Repeat until the vegetables and filling are done.

Nutrition: Calories

31) Spicy cabbage bowl

Preparation time: **Cooking time:**   **Portions:**

Ingredients:
- Sesame seeds (1 tablespoon)
- Green onion (.25 c.)
- Cabbage (2 c.)
- Coconut amino acids (1 teaspoon)
- Tamari (2 tablespoons)
- Chopped kimchi cabbage (1 c.)
- Cooked brown rice (1 c.)
- Chopped garlic (1 teaspoon)
- Grated ginger (.5 tsp.)
- Sesame oil (2 tablespoons)

Directions:
- Take out a frying pan and heat the sesame oil in it. When the oil is hot, add together the coconut amino acid, tamari, kimchi, brown rice, garlic and ginger.
- After five minutes of cooking these ingredients, add the green onions and cabbage and toss to combine.
- Cook for a little longer. Then you can garnish the dish with some sesame seeds before serving.

Nutrition: Calories

32) Citrus and fennel salad

Preparation time: **Cooking time:** **Portions:**

Ingredients:
- ✓ Diced avocado (.5)
- ✓ Pomegranate seeds (2 tablespoons)
- ✓ Pepper (.5 tsp.)
- ✓ Salt (.25 tsp.)
- ✓ Olive oil (.25 c.)
- ✓ Orange juice (2 tablespoons)
- ✓ Lemon juice (2 tablespoons)

Ingredients:
- ✓ Chopped mint (1 tablespoon)
- ✓ Chopped parsley (.5 c.)
- ✓ Sliced fennel bulbs (2)
- ✓ Red grapefruit segmented (.5)
- ✓ Segmented orange (1)

Directions:
- ❖ To start this recipe, bring out a large bowl and combine together the parsley, mint, fennel slices, grapefruit wedges, and orange wedges. Stir to combine.
- ❖ In another bowl, whisk together the pepper, salt, olive oil, orange juice and lemon juice.
- ❖ Once combined, pour over the fennel and citrus mixture in the large bowl, stirring to coat.
- ❖ Move to a plate and garnish with the avocado and pomegranate seeds. Serve immediately.

Nutrition: Calories

33) Vegan Burger

Preparation time: **Cooking time:** **Servings: 4 hamburger patties**

Ingredients:
- ✓ 1/4 to 1/2 cup of spring water
- ✓ 1/2 teaspoon of cayenne powder
- ✓ 1/2 teaspoon of ginger powder
- ✓ Grape oil
- ✓ 1 teaspoon of dill
- ✓ 2 teaspoons of sea salt
- ✓ 2 teaspoons of onion powder

Ingredients:
- ✓ 2 teaspoons of oregano
- ✓ 2 teaspoons of basil
- ✓ ¼ cup cherry tomatoes, diced
- ✓ 1/2 cup of cabbage, diced
- ✓ 1/2 cup green peppers, diced
- ✓ 1/2 cup onions, diced
- ✓ 1 cup of chickpea flour

Directions:
- ❖ Mix the vegetables and seasonings in a large bowl, then add the flour. Gently add the spring water and stir the mixture until combined. If the mixture is too soft, add more flour.
- ❖ Divide the dough into 4 meatballs. Cook patties in grapeseed oil, in a skillet over medium heat for about 2 to 3 minutes per side. Continue flipping until the burger is brown on all sides.
- ❖ Serve the burger on a bun and enjoy.

Nutrition: Calories

34) Alkaline spicy cabbage

Preparation time: **Cooking time:** **Servings: 1 portion**

Ingredients:
- ✓ Grape oil
- ✓ 1/4 teaspoon of sea salt
- ✓ 1 teaspoon crushed red pepper

Ingredients:
- ✓ 1/4 cup red bell bell pepper, diced
- ✓ 1/4 cup onion, diced
- ✓ 1 bunch of cabbage

Directions:
- ❖ First wash the cabbage well and then fold each cabbage leaf in half. Cut off and discard the stems. Cut the prepared cabbage into bite-size portions and use the salad spinner to remove the water.
- ❖ In a wok, add 2 tablespoons of grapeseed oil and heat the oil over high heat.
- ❖ Fry the peppers and onions in the oil for about 2-3 minutes and then season with a little sea salt.
- ❖ Lower the heat and add the cabbage, cover the wok with a lid and simmer for about 5 minutes.
- ❖ Open the lid and add the crushed pepper, mix well and cover again. Cook until tender, or about 3 more minutes.

Nutrition: Calories

35) Electric Salad

Preparation time: **Cooking time:** **Servings: 4**

Ingredients:
- 3 jalapenos
- 2 red onions
- 1 orange bell pepper
- 1 yellow bell pepper
- 1 cup cherry tomatoes, chopped

Ingredients:
- 1 bunch of cabbage
- 1 handful of romaine lettuce
- Extra virgin olive oil
- Juice of 1 lime

Directions:
- First wash and rinse the ingredients well. Dry the ingredients and then cut them into bite-size pieces, or as required.

- Place ingredients in a bowl and drizzle with olive oil and lime juice to your preferred taste.

Nutrition: Calories

36) Kale salad

Preparation time: **Cooking time:** **Servings: 2**

Ingredients:
- 1/4 teaspoon of cayenne
- 1/2 teaspoon of sea salt
- 1/2 cup of cooked chickpeas
- 1/2 cup of red onions
- 1/2 cup sliced red, orange, yellow and green peppers
- 4 cups chopped cabbage

Ingredients:
- 1/2 cup alkaline garlic sauce (recipe included).
- Alkaline Garlic Sauce
- 1/4 teaspoon of dill
- 1/4 teaspoon of sea salt
- 1/2 teaspoon of ginger
- 1 tablespoon of onion powder
- 1/4 cup shallots, chopped
- 1 cup of grape oil

Directions:
- In a bowl, mix all the ingredients for the coleslaw and toss.

- Prepare the dressing by mixing the ingredients for the "Alkaline Electric Garlic Sauce".
- Drizzle with half a cup of sauce and then serve.

Nutrition: Calories

37) Walnut, date, orange and cabbage salad

Preparation time: **Cooking time:** **Servings: 2**

Ingredients:
- /2 red onion, very thinly sliced
- 2 bunches of cabbage, or 6 full cups of sprouts
- 6 medjool dates, pitted
- 1/3 cup whole walnuts
- For the dressing

Ingredients:
- 5 tablespoons of olive oil
- Pinch of coarse salt
- 1 medjool date
- 4 tablespoons of freshly squeezed orange juice
- 2 tablespoons of lime juice

Directions:
- Preheat the oven to 375 degrees F and then place the walnuts on a baking sheet. Roast the walnuts for about 7-8 minutes, or until the skin begins to darken and crack.
- Once done, transfer the walnuts while still warm and let them steam for 15 minutes wrapped in a kitchen towel.
- Once cooled, squeeze and turn firmly to remove the skin, all still wrapped in the towel.
- In a food processor, place the pitted dates along with the walnuts and puree until fully blended and finely chopped. Set aside to cover the salad.

- Then wash, dry and cut the cabbage and place in a large bowl. Thinly slice the onion and add it to the bowl.
- Now prepare the dressing by combining the ingredients for the "dressing" in the blender apart from the olive oil.
- Blend the mixture to break up the dates and then pour in the oil in a steady stream to emulsify the dressing.
- Finally, toss the cabbage and onion mixture with the orange and walnut dressing.
- Move to a serving bowl and sprinkle with the walnut and date mixture. Enjoy!

Nutrition: Calories

38) Tomatoes with basil-snack

Preparation time: **Cooking time:** **Servings: 1 portion**

Ingredients:
- ¼ teaspoon of sea salt
- 2 tablespoons of lemon juice
- 2 tablespoons of olive oil

Ingredients:
- ¼ cup basil, fresh
- 1 cup chopped tomatoes, cherry or Roma

Directions:
- ❖ Start by slicing the cherry tomatoes and placing them in a medium sized bowl.
- ❖ Then finely chop your basil and add it to the bowl of tomatoes.
- ❖ Drizzle the tomatoes and basil with a little olive oil and lemon juice.
- ❖ Add a little sea salt to taste.
- ❖ Serve.

Nutrition: Calories

39) Pasta with spelt, zucchini and eggplant

Preparation time: **Cooking time:** **Servings: 4**

Ingredients:
- 2 teaspoons of dried basil leaves
- 1 teaspoon of oregano
- 2/3 cup vegetable broth
- 2/3 cup of dried and diced cherry tomatoes
- 1 large zucchini, diced
- 3 medium-sized, ripe cherry tomatoes, diced

Ingredients:
- 2-3 ginger, crushed
- 1-2 white onions, finely chopped
- 3 tablespoons of cold-pressed extra virgin olive oil
- 1 large eggplant cut into cubes
- 300g of spelt pasta
- Sea salt to taste

Directions:
- ❖ Over medium heat, heat a little oil in a skillet and then sauté the eggplant, ginger and onion for about 8-10 minutes, stirring constantly.
- ❖ Then add the oregano, tomatoes and zucchini and let cook for 6-8 minutes, stirring occasionally.
- ❖ Now heat the water and cook the pasta until it is firm to the bite, and then add the vegetable broth to the pan.
- ❖ Season with fresh pepper, salt and dried basil. Allow the mixture to simmer for a few minutes, covered.
- ❖ Once cooked, you can serve the sauce over pasta and garnish with fresh basil leaves.

Nutrition: Calories

40) Alkalizing millet dish

Preparation time: **Cooking time:** **Servings: 2**

Ingredients:
- 1/2 teaspoon of sea salt
- 2 1/2 cups of water

Ingredients:
- 1 cup millet

Directions:
- ❖ In a pot with an airtight lid, add the millet and then sauté over medium heat, stirring constantly.
- ❖ As soon as the millet turns golden brown, add the sea salt and water and cover the ingredients with a lid.
- ❖ Then bring the mixture to a boil and let it simmer until all the water has been absorbed, or for about 25-35 minutes.
- ❖ Alternatively, you can cook on an electric stove. Just cover the lid and bring to a boil, simmer for a couple of minutes and then turn off the stove.
- ❖ Allow the contents to cool for about 30 minutes with the lid on to allow the millet to dry out.
- ❖ Then serve and enjoy the millet.

Nutrition: Calories

Chapter 4 -   Dinner Recipes

41) Mixed stew of spicy vegetables

Preparation time: 20 minutes **Cooking time**: 35 minutes **Servings**: 8

Ingredients:
- 2 tablespoons of coconut oil
- 1 large sweet onion, chopped
- 1 medium parsnip, peeled and chopped
- 3 tablespoons of homemade tomato paste
- 2 large garlic cloves, minced
- ½ teaspoon of cinnamon powder
- ½ teaspoon ground ginger
- 1 teaspoon of ground cumin
- ¼ teaspoon cayenne pepper

Directions:
- In a large soup pot, melt the coconut oil over medium-high heat and sauté the onion for about 5 minutes.
- Add the parsnips and sauté for about 3 minutes.
- Add the tomato paste, garlic and spices and sauté for 2 minutes.

Ingredients:
- 2 medium carrots, peeled and chopped
- 2 medium purple potatoes, peeled and cut into pieces
- 2 medium sweet potatoes, peeled and cut into pieces
- 4 cups of homemade vegetable broth
- 2 tablespoons fresh lemon juice
- 2 cups fresh cabbage, hard ribs removed and chopped
- ¼ cup fresh parsley leaves, chopped

- Stir in the carrots, potatoes, sweet potatoes and broth and bring to a boil.
- Reduce heat to medium-low and simmer, covered for about 20 minutes.
- Add the lemon juice and cabbage and simmer for 5 minutes.
- Serve with a garnish of parsley.

Nutrition: Calories

42) Mixed vegetable stew with herbs

Preparation time: 15 minutes **Cooking time**: 2¼ hours **Servings**: 8

Ingredients:
- 2 tablespoons of coconut oil
- 1 medium yellow onion, chopped
- 2 cups celery, chopped
- ½ teaspoon of minced garlic
- 3 cups fresh cabbage, hard ribs removed and chopped
- ½ cup fresh mushrooms, sliced
- 2½ cups tomatoes, finely chopped
- 1 teaspoon dried rosemary, crushed

Directions:
- In a large skillet, melt the coconut oil over medium heat and sauté the onion, celery and garlic for about 5 minutes.
- Add the rest of all ingredients and stir to combine.
- Increase heat to high and bring to a boil.
- Cook for about 10 minutes.

Ingredients:
- 1 teaspoon dried sage, crushed
- 1 teaspoon dried oregano, crushed
- Sea salt and freshly ground black pepper, to taste
- 2 cups of homemade vegetable broth
- 3-4 cups of alkaline water
- ¼ cup fresh parsley, chopped

- Reduce heat to medium and cook, covered for about 15 minutes.
- Uncover the pan and cook for about 15 minutes, stirring occasionally.
- Now, reduce the heat to low and simmer, covered for about 1 1/2 hours.
- Serve warm with a garnish of parsley.

Nutrition: Calories

43) Tofu and bell pepper stew

Preparation time: 15 minutes **Cooking time**: 15 minutes **Servings**: 6

Ingredients:
- 2 tablespoons of garlic
- 1 jalapeño bell pepper, seeded and chopped
- 1 (16-ounce) can of roasted, rinsed, drained and chopped red peppers
- 2 cups of homemade vegetable broth
- 2 cups of alkaline water

Directions:
- In a food processor, add the garlic, jalapeño bell pepper and roasted red peppers and pulse until smooth.
- In a large skillet, add the pepper puree, broth and water over medium-high heat and bring to a boil.
- Add the peppers and tofu and stir to combine.

Nutrition: Calories

Ingredients:
- 1 medium green bell pepper, seeded and thinly sliced
- 1 medium red bell pepper, seeded and thinly sliced
- 1 (16-ounce) package of extra-firm tofu, drained and diced
- 10 ounces of frozen sprouts, thawed
- Sea salt and freshly ground black pepper, to taste

- Reduce the heat to medium and cook for about 5 minutes.
- Stir in the cabbage and cook for about 5 minutes.
- Add the salt and black pepper and remove from heat.
- Serve hot.

44) Roasted Pumpkin Curry

Preparation time: 15 minutes **Cooking time**: 35 minutes **Servings**: 4

Ingredients:
For the roasted squash:
- ✓ 1 medium-sized sugar pumpkin, peeled and cut into cubes
- ✓ Sea salt, to taste
- ✓ 1 teaspoon of olive oil

For Curry:
- ✓ 1 teaspoon of olive oil
- ✓ 1 onion, chopped
- ✓ 1 tablespoon fresh ginger root, peeled and chopped

Directions:
- ❖ Preheat oven to 400 degrees F. Line a large baking sheet with baking paper.
- ❖ In a large bowl, add all the ingredients for the roasted squash and stir to coat well.
- ❖ Arrange the pumpkins on the prepared baking sheet in a single layer.
- ❖ Roast for about 20-25 minutes, turning once halfway through.

Ingredients:
- ✓ 1 tablespoon chopped garlic
- ✓ 1 cup unsweetened coconut milk
- ✓ 2 cups of vegetable broth
- ✓ 1 teaspoon of ground cumin
- ✓ ½ teaspoon ground turmeric
- ✓ Sea salt and freshly ground black pepper, to taste
- ✓ 1 tablespoon fresh lime juice
- ✓ 2 tablespoons fresh parsley, chopped
- ❖ Meanwhile, for the curry: in a large skillet, heat the oil over medium-high heat and sauté the onion for about 4-5 minutes.
- ❖ Add the ginger and garlic and sauté for about 1 minute.
- ❖ Add the coconut milk, broth, spices, salt and black pepper and bring to a boil.
- ❖ Reduce the heat to low and simmer for about 10 minutes.
- ❖ Add the roasted squash and simmer for another 10 minutes.
- ❖ Serve warm with a garnish of parsley.

Nutrition: Calories

45) Lentils, vegetables and apple curry

Preparation time: 20 minutes **Cooking time:** 1 hour and a half **Servings:** 6

Ingredients:
- ✓ 8 cups of alkaline water
- ✓ ½ teaspoon ground turmeric
- ✓ 1 cup brown lentils
- ✓ 1 cup of red lentils
- ✓ 1 tablespoon of olive oil
- ✓ 1 large white onion, chopped
- ✓ 3 garlic cloves, minced
- ✓ 2 tomatoes, seeded and chopped

Directions:
- ❖ In a large skillet, add the water, turmeric and lentils over high heat and bring to a boil.
- ❖ Reduce heat to medium-low and simmer, covered for about 30 minutes.
- ❖ Drain the lentils, reserving 2½ cups of the cooking liquid.
- ❖ Meanwhile, in another large skillet, heat the oil over medium heat and sauté the onion for about 2-3 minutes.
- ❖ Add the garlic and sauté for about 1 minute.
- ❖ Add the tomatoes and cook for about 5 minutes.

Ingredients:
- ✓ ¼ teaspoon ground cloves
- ✓ 2 teaspoons of ground cumin
- ✓ 2 carrots, peeled and cut into pieces
- ✓ 2 potatoes, peeled and cut into pieces
- ✓ 2 cups pumpkin, peeled, seeded and cut into 1-inch cubes
- ✓ 1 granny smith apple, cored and chopped
- ✓ 2 cups fresh cabbage, hard ribs removed and chopped
- ✓ Sea salt and freshly ground black pepper, to taste
- ❖ Stir in the spices and cook for about 1 minute.
- ❖ Add the carrots, potatoes, squash, cooked lentils and reserved cooking liquid and bring to a gentle boil.
- ❖ Reduce heat to medium-low and simmer, covered for about 40-45 minutes or until desired doneness of vegetables.
- ❖ Add the apple and cabbage and simmer for about 15 minutes.
- ❖ Add the salt and black pepper and remove from heat.
- ❖ Serve hot.

Nutrition: Calories

46) Curried red beans

Preparation time: 15 minutes **Cooking time:** 25 minutes **Servings:** 6

Ingredients:
- ✓ 4 tablespoons of olive oil
- ✓ 1 medium onion, finely chopped
- ✓ 2 garlic cloves, minced
- ✓ 2 tablespoons of fresh ginger root, peeled and chopped
- ✓ 1 teaspoon of ground coriander
- ✓ 1 teaspoon of ground cumin
- ✓ ½ teaspoon ground turmeric

Directions:
- ❖ In a large skillet, heat the oil over medium heat and sauté the onion, garlic and ginger for about 6-8 minutes.
- ❖ Stir in the spices and cook for about 1-2 minutes.

Ingredients:
- ✓ ¼ teaspoon cayenne pepper
- ✓ Sea salt and freshly ground black pepper, to taste
- ✓ 2 large plum tomatoes, finely chopped
- ✓ 3 cups of cooked red beans
- ✓ 2 cups of alkaline water
- ✓ ¼ cup fresh parsley, chopped
- ❖ Add the tomatoes, beans and water and bring to a boil over high heat.
- ❖ Reduce heat to medium and simmer for 10-15 minutes or until desired thickness.
- ❖ Serve warm with a garnish of parsley.

Nutrition: Calories

47) Lentil and Carrot Chili

Preparation time: 15 minutes **Cooking time:** 2 hours and 40 minutes **Servings:** 8

Ingredients:
- 2 teaspoons of olive oil
- 1 large onion, chopped
- 3 medium carrots, peeled and chopped
- 4 celery stalks, chopped
- 2 garlic cloves, minced
- • 1 jalapeño bell pepper, seeded and chopped
- ½ tablespoon dried thyme, crushed
- 1 tablespoon of chipotle chili powder

Directions:
- In a large skillet, heat the oil over medium heat and sauté the onion, carrot and celery for about 5 minutes.
- Add the garlic, jalapeño pepper, thyme and spices and sauté for about 1 minute.

Nutrition: Calories

Ingredients:
- ½ tablespoon of cayenne pepper
- 1½ tablespoons ground coriander
- 1½ tablespoons of ground cumin
- 1 teaspoon ground turmeric
- Sea salt and freshly ground black pepper, to taste
- 1 pound red lentils, rinsed
- 8 cups of homemade vegetable broth
- ½ cup shallots, chopped

- Add the lentils and broth and bring to a boil.
- Reduce heat to low and simmer, covered for about 2-2½ hours.
- Remove from heat and serve hot with a scallion garnish.

48) Black beans with chilli

Preparation time: 15 minutes **Cooking time:** 2 hours and 5 minutes **Servings:** 5

Ingredients:
- 2 tablespoons of olive oil
- 1 onion, chopped
- 1 large green bell pepper, seeded and sliced
- 4 garlic cloves, minced
- 2 jalapeño peppers, sliced
- 1 teaspoon of ground cumin
- 1 teaspoon of cayenne pepper

Directions:
- In a large skillet, heat the oil over medium-high heat and sauté the onion and peppers for 3-4 minutes.
- Add the garlic, jalapeño peppers and spices and sauté for about 1 minute.
- Add the remaining ingredients and bring to a boil.

Nutrition: Calories

Ingredients:
- 1 tablespoon of red chili powder
- 1 teaspoon of paprika
- 2 cups of tomatoes, finely chopped
- 4 cups of cooked black beans
- 2 cups of homemade vegetable broth
- Sea salt and freshly ground black pepper, to taste
- ¼ cup fresh parsley, chopped

- Reduce heat to medium-low and simmer, covered for about 1½-2 hours.
- Season with the salt and black pepper and remove from heat.
- Serve warm with a garnish of parsley.

49) Cook mixed vegetables

Preparation time: 15 minutes **Cooking time:** 20 minutes **Servings:** 4

Ingredients:
- 1 small zucchini, chopped
- 1 small summer squash, chopped
- 1 diced eggplant
- 1 red bell pepper, seeded and diced
- 1 green bell pepper, seeded and diced

Directions:
- Preheat oven to 375 degrees F. Lightly grease a large baking dish.
- In a large bowl, add all ingredients and mix well.

Nutrition: Calories

Ingredients:
- 1 onion, thinly sliced
- 1 tablespoon of pure maple syrup
- 2 tablespoons of olive oil
- Sea salt and freshly ground black pepper, to taste

- Transfer the vegetable mixture to the prepared baking dish.
- Bake for about 15-20 minutes.
- Remove from oven and serve immediately.

50) Vegetarian Ratatouille

Preparation time: 20 minutes **Cooking time:** 45 minutes **Servings:** 4

Ingredients:
- 6 ounces of homemade tomato paste
- 3 tablespoons of olive oil, divided by
- ½ onion, chopped
- 3 tablespoons minced garlic
- Sea salt and freshly ground black pepper, to taste
- 1 zucchini, cut into thin circles

Directions:
- Preheat the oven to 375 degrees F.
- In a bowl, add tomato paste, 1 tablespoon oil, onion, garlic, salt and black pepper and mix well.
- In the bottom of a 10x10-inch baking dish, spread tomato paste mixture evenly.

Ingredients:
- 1 yellow pumpkin, cut in thin circles
- 1 eggplant, cut into thin circles
- 1 red bell pepper, with seeds and cut into thin rounds
- 1 yellow bell pepper, with seeds and cut into thin rounds
- 1 tablespoon fresh thyme leaves, chopped
- 1 tablespoon fresh lemon juice

- Drizzle the vegetables with the remaining oil and sprinkle with salt and black pepper, followed by the thyme.
- Arrange a piece of parchment paper over the vegetables.
- Bake for about 45 minutes.
- Remove from oven and serve hot.

- ❖ Arrange the vegetable slices alternately, starting at the outer edge of the pan and working concentrically toward the center.

Nutrition: Calories

51) Quinoa with vegetables

Preparation time: 15 minutes **Cooking time**: 26 minutes **Servings**: 4

Ingredients:
- For roasted mushrooms:
- ✓ 2 cups of small fresh Baby Bella mushrooms
- ✓ 1 tablespoon of olive oil
- ✓ Sea salt, to taste
- For the quinoa:
- ✓ 2 cups of alkaline water
- ✓ 1 cup red quinoa, rinsed
- ✓ 2 tablespoons fresh parsley, chopped

Directions:
- ❖ Preheat oven to 425 degrees F. Line a large rimmed baking sheet with parchment paper.
- ❖ In a bowl, add the mushrooms, oil and salt and stir to coat well.
- ❖ Arrange the mushrooms on the prepared baking sheet in a single layer.
- ❖ Roast for about 15-18 minutes, tossing once halfway through cooking.
- ❖ Meanwhile, for the quinoa: in a skillet, add the water and quinoa over medium-high heat and bring to a boil.
- ❖ Reduce the heat to low and simmer, covered for about 15-20 minutes or until all the liquid is absorbed.
- ❖ Remove from heat and set pan aside, covered for about 5 minutes.
- ❖ Uncover the pan and with a fork, stir in the quinoa.

Ingredients:
- ✓ 1 garlic clove chopped
- ✓ 1 tablespoon of olive oil
- ✓ 2 teaspoons of fresh lemon juice
- ✓ Sea salt and freshly ground black pepper, to taste
- For the broccoli:
- ✓ 1 cup of broccoli florets
- ✓ 2 tablespoons of olive oil

- ❖ Stir in the parsley, garlic, oil, lemon juice, salt and black pepper and set aside to cool completely.
- ❖ Meanwhile, for the broccoli: in a pot of water, arrange a steamer basket and bring to a boil.
- ❖ Place the broccoli florets in the basket of the steamer and steam, covered for about 5-6 minutes.
- ❖ Drain broccoli florets well.
- ❖ Transfer the broccoli florets to the bowl with the quinoa and mushrooms and stir to combine.
- ❖ Drizzle with the oil and serve immediately.

Nutrition: Calories

52) Lentils with cabbage

Preparation time: 15 minutes **Cooking time**: 20 minutes **Servings**: 6

Ingredients:
- ✓ 1½ cups of red lentils
- ✓ 1½ cups homemade vegetable broth
- ✓ 1½ tablespoons of olive oil
- ✓ ½ cup onion, chopped
- ✓ 1 teaspoon fresh ginger, chopped

Directions:
- ❖ In a skillet, add the broth and lentils over medium-high heat and bring to a boil.
- ❖ Reduce heat and simmer, covered for about 20 minutes or until almost all liquid is absorbed.
- ❖ Remove from heat and set aside covered.

Nutrition: Calories

Ingredients:
- ✓ 2 garlic cloves, minced
- ✓ 1½ cups tomato, chopped
- ✓ 6 cups fresh cabbage, hard ribs removed and chopped
- ✓ Sea salt and ground black pepper, to taste

- ❖ Meanwhile, in a large skillet, heat the oil over medium heat and sauté the onion for about 5-6 minutes.
- ❖ Add the ginger and garlic and sauté for about 1 minute.
- ❖ Add the tomatoes and cabbage and cook for about 4-5 minutes.
- ❖ Add the lentils, salt and black pepper and remove from heat.
- ❖ Remove from heat and serve hot.

53) Lentils with tomatoes

Preparation time: 15 minutes   **Cooking time**: 55 minutes   **Servings**: 4

Ingredients:
- For the tomato puree:
- 1 cup tomatoes, chopped
- 1 garlic clove, minced
- 1 green chilli chopped
- ¼ cup alkaline water
- For the lentils:
- 1 cup of red lentils
- 3 cups of alkaline water

Ingredients:
- 1 tablespoon of olive oil
- ½ medium white onion, chopped
- ½ teaspoon of ground cumin
- ½ teaspoon of cayenne pepper
- ¼ teaspoon ground turmeric
- ¼ cup tomato, chopped
- ¼ cup fresh parsley leaves, chopped

Directions:
- To tomato paste in a blender, add all ingredients and pulse until it forms a smooth puree. Set aside.
- In a large skillet, add 3 cups of water and the lentils over high heat and bring to a boil.
- Reduce heat to medium-low and simmer, covered for about 15-20 minutes or until quite tender.
- Drain lentils well.
- In a large skillet, heat the oil over medium heat and sauté the onion for about 6-7 minutes.
- Add the spices and sauté for about 1 minute.
- Add the tomato puree and cook, stirring for about 5-7 minutes.
- Stir in lentils and cook for about 4-5 minutes or until desired degree of doneness.
- Stir in chopped tomato and immediately remove from heat.
- Serve warm with a garnish of parsley.

Nutrition: Calories

54) Spicy baked beans

Preparation time: 15 minutes   **Cooking time**: 2 hours and 5 minutes   **Servings**: 4

Ingredients:
- ½ pound of dried red beans, soaked overnight and drained
- 1¼ tablespoons of olive oil
- 1 small yellow onion, chopped
- 4 garlic cloves, minced
- 1 teaspoon dried thyme, crushed
- ½ teaspoon of ground cumin
- ½ teaspoon of red pepper flakes, crushed

Ingredients:
- ¼ teaspoon of smoked paprika
- 1 tablespoon fresh lemon juice
- 1 cup of homemade tomato sauce
- 1 cup of homemade vegetable broth
- Sea salt and freshly ground black pepper, to taste

Directions:
- In a large pot of boiling water, add the beans and bring to a boil.
- Reduce heat to low and cook, covered for about 1 hour.
- Remove from heat and drain beans well.
- Preheat the oven to 325 degrees F.
- In a large ovenproof skillet, heat the oil over medium heat and sauté the onion for about 4 minutes.
- Add the garlic, thyme and spices and sauté for about 1 minute.
- Add the cooked beans and other ingredients and immediately remove from heat.
- Cover the pan and bake for about 1 hour.
- Remove from oven and serve hot.

Nutrition: Calories

55) Chickpeas with pumpkin

Preparation time: 20 minutes   **Cooking time**: 35 minutes   **Servings**: 4

Ingredients:
- 1 tablespoon of olive oil
- 1 onion, chopped
- 2 garlic cloves, minced
- 1 green chili pepper, seedless and finely chopped
- 1 teaspoon of ground cumin
- ½ teaspoon of ground coriander
- 1 teaspoon of red chili powder

Directions:
- In a large skillet, heat the oil over medium-high heat and sauté the onion for about 5-7 minutes.
- Add the garlic, green chiles and spices and sauté for about 1 minute.
- Add tomatoes and cook for 2-3 minutes, mashing with the back of a spoon.

Ingredients:
- 2 cups fresh tomatoes, finely chopped
- 2 pounds of pumpkin, peeled and diced
- 2 cups of homemade vegetable broth
- 2 cups of cooked chickpeas
- 2 tablespoons fresh lemon juice
- Sea salt and freshly ground black pepper, to taste
- 2 tablespoons fresh parsley leaves, chopped
- Add the squash and cook for about 3-4 minutes, stirring occasionally.
- Add the broth and bring to a boil.
- Reduce the heat to low and simmer for about 10 minutes.
- Stir in the chickpeas and simmer for about 10 minutes.
- Add the lemon juice, salt and black pepper and remove from heat.
- Serve warm with a garnish of parsley.

Nutrition: Calories

56) Chickpeas with cabbage

Preparation time: 15 minutes   **Cooking time**: 18 minutes   **Servings**: 6

Ingredients:
- 2 tablespoons of olive oil
- 1 medium onion, chopped
- 4 garlic cloves, minced
- 1 teaspoon dried thyme, crushed
- 1 teaspoon dried oregano, crushed
- ½ teaspoon of paprika
- 1 cup of tomato, finely chopped

Directions:
- In a large skillet, heat the oil over medium heat and sauté the onion for about 8-9 minutes.
- Add the garlic, herbs and paprika and sauté for about 1 minute.
- Add the cabbage and water and cook for about 2-3 minutes.

Nutrition: Calories

Ingredients:
- 2 ½ cups cooked chickpeas
- 4 cups fresh cabbage, hard ribs removed and chopped
- 2 tablespoons of alkaline water
- 2 tablespoons fresh lemon juice
- Sea salt and freshly ground black pepper, to taste
- 3 tablespoons fresh basil, chopped

- Add the tomatoes and chickpeas and cook for about 3-5 minutes.
- Add the lemon juice, salt and black pepper and remove from heat.
- Serve warm with the basil garnish.

57) Stuffed cabbage rolls

Preparation time: 15 minutes **Cooking time:** 15 minutes **Servings:** 4

Ingredients:
For filling:
- 1½ cups fresh button mushrooms, chopped
- 3¼ cups zucchini, chopped
- 1 cup red bell bell pepper, seeded and chopped
- 1 cup green bell pepper, seeded and chopped
- ½ teaspoon dried thyme, crushed
- ½ teaspoon dried marjoram, crushed
- ½ teaspoon dried basil, crushed

Directions:
- Preheat oven to 400 degrees F. Lightly grease a 13x9-inch casserole dish.
- For the filling: in a large skillet, add all ingredients except lemon juice over medium heat and bring to a boil.
- Reduce heat to low and simmer, covered for about 5 minutes.
- Remove from heat and set aside for about 5 minutes.
- Add the lemon juice and stir to combine.
- Meanwhile, for the rolls: in a large pot of boiling water, add the cabbage leaves and boil for about 2-4 minutes.
- Drain the cabbage leaves well.
- Thoroughly dry each cabbage leaf with paper towels.
- Arrange the cabbage leaves on a smooth surface.
- Using a knife, make a V-shaped cut in each leaf by cutting through the thick vein.

Nutrition: Calories

Ingredients:
- Sea salt and freshly ground black pepper, to taste
- ½ cup homemade vegetable broth
- 2 teaspoons of fresh lemon juice
For rolls:
- 8 large cabbage leaves, rinsed
- 8 ounces of homemade tomato sauce
- 3 tablespoons fresh parsley, chopped

- Carefully overlap the cut ends of each leaf.
- Place the filling mixture evenly on each leaf and fold in the sides.
- Then, roll up each leaf to seal in the filling and then, secure each leaf with toothpicks.
- In the bottom of the prepared casserole dish, place 1/3 cup of the tomato sauce evenly.
- Arrange cabbage rolls on top of sauce in a single layer and top with remaining sauce evenly.
- Cover the casserole dish and cook for about 15 minutes.
- Remove from oven and set aside, uncovered for about 5 minutes.
- Serve warm with a garnish of parsley.

58) Green beans and mushrooms in casserole

Preparation time: 20 minutes **Cooking time:** 20 minutes **Servings:** 6

Ingredients:
- For the onion slices:
- ½ cup yellow onion, very thinly sliced
- ¼ cup almond flour
- 1/8 teaspoon of garlic powder
- Sea salt and freshly ground black pepper, to taste
- For the casserole:
- 1 pound fresh green beans, chopped
- 1 tablespoon of olive oil

Directions:
- Preheat the oven to 350 degrees F.
- For the onion slices: in a bowl, place all ingredients and mix to coat well.
- Arrange the onion slices on a large baking sheet in a single layer and set aside.
- For the casserole: in a pot of boiling salted water, add the green beans and cook for about 5 minutes.
- Drain green beans and transfer to a bowl of ice water.
- Again, drain well and transfer to a large bowl. Set aside.
- In a large skillet, heat the oil over medium-high heat and sauté the mushrooms, onion, garlic powder, salt and black pepper for about 2-3 minutes.

Nutrition: Calories

Ingredients:
- 8 ounces fresh cremini mushrooms, sliced
- ½ cup yellow onion, thinly sliced
- 1/8 teaspoon of garlic powder
- Sea salt and freshly ground black pepper, to taste
- 1 teaspoon fresh thyme, chopped
- ½ cup homemade vegetable broth
- ½ cup of coconut cream

- Stir in the thyme and broth and cook for about 3-5 minutes or until all the liquid is absorbed.
- Remove from heat and transfer the mushroom mixture to the bowl with the green beans.
- Add the coconut cream and stir to combine well.
- Transfer the mixture to a 10-inch casserole dish.
- Place the casserole dish and onion slice pan in the oven.
- Bake for about 15-17 minutes.
- Remove the pan and sheet from the oven and let cool for about 5 minutes before serving.
- Top the casserole with the crispy onion slices evenly.
- Cut into 6 equal-sized portions and serve.

59) Meatloaf of wild rice and lentils

Preparation time: 20 minutes **Cooking time:** 1 hour and 50 minutes **Servings:** 8

Ingredients:
- 1¾ cups plus 2 tablespoons of alkaline water, divided
- ½ cup wild rice
- ½ cup of brown lentils
- Pinch of sea salt
- ½ teaspoon of sodium-free Italian seasoning
- 1 medium yellow onion, chopped
- 1 celery stalk, chopped
- 6 cremini mushrooms, chopped

Directions:
- In a saucepan, add 1¾ cups water, the rice, lentils, salt and Italian seasoning and bring to a boil over medium-high heat.
- Reduce the heat to low and simmer covered for about 45 minutes.
- Remove from heat and set aside, covered for at least 10 minutes.
- Preheat oven to 350 degrees F. Line a 9x5-inch baking dish with baking paper.
- In a skillet, heat the remaining water over medium heat and sauté the onion, celery, mushrooms and garlic for about 4-5 minutes.
- Remove from heat and allow to cool slightly.
- In a large bowl, add the oats, pecans, tomato sauce and fresh herbs and stir until well combined.

Nutrition: Calories

Ingredients:
- 4 garlic cloves, minced
- ¾ cup rolled oats
- ½ cup pecans, finely chopped
- ¾ cup of homemade tomato sauce
- ½ teaspoon of red pepper flakes, crushed
- 1 teaspoon fresh rosemary, chopped
- 2 teaspoons fresh thyme, chopped

- Combine the rice mixture and vegetable mixture with the oat mixture and mix well.
- In a blender, add the mixture and pulse until it forms a chunky mixture.
- Transfer the mixture to the prepared baking dish evenly.
- With a piece of foil, cover the pan and bake for about 40 minutes.
- Uncover and bake for about 15-20 minutes more or until the top turns golden brown.
- Remove from oven and set aside for about 5-10 minutes before slicing.
- Cut into slices of desired size and serve

60) *Vegetable soup and spelt noodles*

Preparation time: 5 minutes **Cooking time**: 12 minutes **Servings: 2**

Ingredients:
- ½ onion, peeled, cut into cubes
- ½ green bell pepper, chopped
- ½ zucchini, grated
- 4 ounces (113 g) sliced mushrooms, chopped
- ½ cup of cherry tomatoes
- ¼ cup of basil leaves

Directions:
- Take a medium saucepan, put it over medium heat, add the oil and when hot, add the onion and then cook for 3 minutes or more until tender.
- Add the cherry tomatoes, bell bell pepper and mushrooms, stir until combined and continue cooking for 3 minutes until soft.
- Add the grated zucchini, season with salt, cayenne pepper, pour in the water and bring the mixture to a boil.

Nutrition: Calories

Ingredients:
- 1 package of spelt tagliatelle, cooked
- ¼ teaspoon salt
- ⅛ teaspoon of cayenne pepper
- ½ key lime, squeezed
- 1 tablespoon of grape oil
- 2 cups of spring water

- Then, turn the heat down to low, add the cooked noodles and simmer the soup for 5 minutes.
- When finished, pour soup into two bowls, top with basil leaves, drizzle with lime juice and serve.

Chapter 5 - Snacks Recipes

61) Quinoa Salad

Preparation time: **Cooking time:** **Servings: 2**

Ingredients:
- ✓ 1 cup quinoa, cooked
- ✓ 1 garlic clove, minced
- ✓ 1 cucumber, chopped
- ✓ 1 cup of fresh arugula leaves
- ✓ 1 red bell pepper, chopped
- ✓ 1 large avocado, peeled, pitted and diced

Directions:
- ❖ Just combine all the ingredients in a large salad bowl.

Nutrition: Calories

Ingredients:
- ✓ 2 tablespoons of chia seeds (optional)
- ✓ 2 tablespoons of olive oil
- ✓ 2 tablespoons of coconut milk (I think)
- ✓ Himalayan salt and black pepper to taste
- ✓ Juice of 1 lime or lemon

- ❖ Mix well and drizzle with olive oil, coconut milk and lemon juice.
- ❖ Enjoy!

62) Almonds with sautéed vegetables

Preparation time: **Cooking time:** **Servings: 4**

Ingredients:
- ✓ Young beans, 150g
- ✓ Broccoli flower, 4
- ✓ Oregano and cumin, ½ teaspoon
- ✓ Lemon juice (fresh), 3 tablespoons
- ✓ Garlic clove (finely chopped), 1

Directions:
- ❖ Add broccoli, beans and other vegetables to a large skillet and fry until beans and broccoli turn dark green.
- ❖ Make sure the vegetables are crispy as well.
- ❖ Now add the chopped garlic and onion, sauté and stir for a few minutes.

Nutrition: Calories

Ingredients:
- ✓ Cauliflower, 1 cup
- ✓ Olive oil (cold pressed), 4 tablespoons
- ✓ Pepper and salt to taste
- ✓ Some soaked almonds (sliced), for garnish
- ✓ Yellow onion, 1

- ❖ Then, put the dressing together.
- ❖ Take a small bowl, add the lemon juice, oregano, cumin and oil and mix well.
- ❖ Add some vegetables, stir slowly and taste for pepper and salt.
- ❖ Finally, use the sliced almonds for garnish.
- ❖ Serve.

63) Alkaline Sweet Potato Mash

Preparation time: **Cooking time:** **Servings: 3-4**

Ingredients:
- ✓ Sea salt, 1 tablespoon
- ✓ Curry powder, ½ tablespoon
- ✓ Sweet potatoes (large), 6

Directions:
- ❖ First, get a large mixing bowl.
- ❖ Wash and cut the sweet potatoes and add them to the cooking pot and cook for about twenty minutes.

Nutrition: Calories

Ingredients:
- ✓ Coconut milk (fresh), 1 ½ - 2 cups
- ✓ Extra virgin olive oil (cold pressed), 1 tablespoon
- ✓ Pepper, 1 pinch

- ❖ Then, remove the sweet potatoes and mash them to your desired consistency.
- ❖ Finally, all you have to do is add the remaining ingredients and serve.

64) Mediterranean peppers

Preparation time: **Cooking time:** **Servings: 2**

Ingredients:
- ✓ Oregano, 1 teaspoon
- ✓ Garlic cloves (crushed), 2
- ✓ Fresh parsley (chopped), 2 tablespoons
- ✓ Vegetable broth (no yeast), 1 cup
- ✓ Provincial herbs, 1 teaspoon

Directions:
- ❖ Heat the olive oil in a skillet over medium heat, add the bell bell pepper and onions and stir.
- ❖ Add the garlic and stir.

Nutrition: Calories

Ingredients:
- ✓ Red bell pepper (sliced) 2 + Yellow bell pepper (sliced) 2
- ✓ Red onions (thinly sliced), 2 medium-sized
- ✓ Extra virgin olive oil (cold pressed), 2 tablespoons
- ✓ Salt and pepper to taste

- ❖ Then, add the vegetable stock and season with parsley and herbs, as well as pepper and salt to taste.
- ❖ Cover the pan and let it cook for fourteen to fifteen minutes.
- ❖ Serve.

65) Tomato and avocado sauce with potatoes

Preparation time: **Cooking time:**   **Servings: 3**

Ingredients:
- Red onion 1
- 2 Tomatoes
- ½ - 1 lemon (squeezed)
- Chives (fresh and chopped), 1 teaspoon
- Parsley (fresh and chopped), 1 teaspoon

Directions:
- Take a pan and cook the potatoes in salted water, (cook the potatoes with the skin intact).
- Next, peel the avocado, toss it in a bowl and mash it with a fork.

Nutrition: Calories

Ingredients:
- Cayenne pepper, ½ teaspoon
- Avocado (ripe), 2
- Waxy potatoes (medium size), 6
- Saltwater
- Pepper and salt
- Now, dice the onion and tomatoes, add them to the bowl along with the parsley, chives and cayenne.
- Mix well and season with pepper, lemon juice and salt.
- Serve along with the potatoes.

66) Alkaline beans and coconut

Preparation time: **Cooking time:**   **Servings: 4**

Ingredients:
- Ground cumin, ½ teaspoon
- Red chili pepper (chopped), 1-2
- Coconut milk (fresh), 3 tablespoons
- Dry flaked coconut, 1 tablespoon
- Garlic (chopped), 2 cloves
- Cayenne pepper, 1 pinch

Directions:
- Heat the oil in a skillet and add the beans, cumin, garlic, ginger and glaze and sauté for about six minutes.

Nutrition: Calories

Ingredients:
- Sea salt, 1 pinch
- Extra virgin olive oil (cold pressed), 3 tablespoons
- Fresh herbs of your choice, 1 teaspoon
- One (1) pound of green beans, cut into 1-inch pieces
- Fresh ginger (chopped), ½ teaspoon

- Add the coconut flakes and oil and sauté until the milk is fully cooked (this may take three or four minutes).
- Season with pepper, salt and herbs to taste. Serve.

67) Alkalized vegetable lasagna

Preparation time: **Cooking time:**   **Servings: 1**

Ingredients:
- Parsley root, 1
- Leek (small), 1
- Radish (small), 1
- Corn salad, 1
- Tomatoes (large), 3
- Garlic, 1 clove

Directions:
- Take a blender and add the lemon juice, garlic clove and avocado.
- Cut the bell bell pepper into thin strips, cut the leek into thin rings and finely grate the parsley root and radish. When you are done, mix everything with the avocado cream.

Nutrition: Calories

Ingredients:
- Avocado (soft), 2
- Lemon (squeezed), 1-2
- Arugula, 1
- Parsley (few)
- Red bell pepper, 1

- Let's start with the first layer of the lasagna.
- Deposit corn salad in a casserole dish, add avocado spread well.
- For the second layer, add the sliced tomatoes.
- Finally, add the arugula and parsley for the final layer.
- Serve.

68) Aloo Gobi

Preparation time: **Cooking time**:   **Servings**: 1 bowl

Ingredients:
- Cauliflower, 750g
- Fresh ginger, 20g
- Large onions, 2
- Mint, 1/3 cup
- Turmeric, 2 teaspoons
- Diced tomatoes, 400g
- Fresh garlic, 2 cloves
- Cayenne pepper, 2 teaspoons

Ingredients:
- Cilantro/coriander leaves, 1/3 cup
- Large potatoes, 4
- Garam masala, 2 teaspoons
- Green chilli, 4
- Water, 3 cups
- Extra virgin olive oil (cold pressed), 125 ml
- Salt to taste

Directions:
- Blend the chili, garlic and ginger.
- Fry oil in a wok for three minutes and add onion until golden brown.
- Add ground pasta and sauté for a few seconds, then add; garam masala, chili, turmeric, tomatoes and salt.
- Cook for about five minutes and add all other ingredients.
- Stir for three minutes and add the water.
- Cook until sauce is thick.
- Serve with Basmati rice or as a side dish.

Nutrition: Calories

69) Chocolate Crunch Bars

Preparation time: 3 hours   **Cooking time**: 5 minutes   **Servings**: 4

Ingredients:
- 1 1/2 cups sugar-free chocolate chips
- 1 cup of nut butter
- Stevia for taste

Ingredients:
- 1/4 cup of coconut oil
- 3 cups pecans, chopped

Directions:
- Prepare an 8-inch baking dish with baking paper.
- Mix chips chocolate with butter, coconut oil and sweetener in a bowl.
- Melt in the microwave for 2 to 3 minutes until melted.
- Add the nut and nuts. Stir gently.
- Put this wand in the oven and then it won't open anymore.
- Refrigerate for 2 to 3 hours.
- Slice and serve.

Nutrition: Calories 316 Fat: 30.9g. Carbs: 8.3g. Protein: 6.4g. Fiber: 3.8g.

70) Nut Butter Bars

Preparation time: 40 minutes.   **Cooking time**: 10 minutes.   **Servings**: 6

Ingredients:
- 3/4 cup of walnut flour
- 2 ounces of nut butter
- 1/4 cup Swerve

Ingredients:
- 1/2 wooden walnut
- 1/2 teaspoon vanilla

Directions:
- Combine all the ingredients for best results.
- Transfer contents to a small 6-inch baking dish. Press down firmly.
- Refrigerate for 30 minutes.
- Cut into slices and serve.

Nutrition: Calories 214 Fat: 19g. Carbs: 6.5g. Protein: 6.5g. Fiber: 2.1g.

71) Homemade Protein Bar

Preparation time: 5 mnutes   **Cooking time**: 10 minutes   **Servings**: 4

Ingredients:
- 1 knob of butter
- 4 tablespoons of coconut oil
- 2 scoops of vanilla protein

Ingredients:
- To taste, ½ teaspoon of sea salt Optional Ingredients:
- 1 teaspoon cinnamon

Directions:
- Mix coconut oil with butter, protein, stevia and salt in a dish.
- Mix cinnamon and chocolate chips.
- Presss the dough is firmly and freeze until firmed.
- Cut the crust into small bars.
- Serve and enjoy.

Nutrition: Calories 179 Fat: 15.7g. Carbohydrates: 4.8g. Protein: 5.6g. Fiber: 0.8g.

72) Shortbread Coookies

Preparation time: 10 minutes   **Cooking time**: 1 hour and 10 minutes   **Servings**: 6

Ingredients:
- 2 1/2 cups coconut flour
- 6 tablespoons of nut butter

Directions:
- Preheat our oven to 350 degrees.
- Place on a cookie sheet with the parchment paper.
- Beat the butter with the erythritol until fluffy.
- Add the vanilla essence and coconut flour.

Ingredients:
- 1/2 cup erythritol
- 1 teaspoon of vanilla essence

- Mix everything together until crumbly.
- Spoon out a tablespoon of cookie dough onto the cookie sheet.
- Add more dough to make a stack.
- Bake for 15 minutes until golden brown.
- Serve.

Nutrition: Calories 288 Fat: 25.3g. Carbohydrates: 9.6g. Protein: 7.6g. Fiber: 3.8g.

73) Coconut cookies Chip

Preparation time: 10 minutes   **Cooking time:** 15 minutes   **Servings:** 4

Ingredients:
- 1 cup of walnut flour
- ½ cup cacao nibs
- ½ cup coconut flakes, unsweetened
- 1/3 cup erythritol
- ½ cup nut butter

Directions:
- Prepare the oven for 350 degrees F.
- Layer a cookie sheet with parchment paper.
- Add and combine all ingredients dry in a glass bowl.
- Coconut milk, coconut milk, vanilla, stevia and peanut butter.
- Beating well compared to stir in the battery. Mix well.

Ingredients:
- ¼ cup peanut launcher, more than once
- ¼ cup of coconut milk
- Stevia, to taste
- ¼ teaspoon of sea salt

- Spoon out a tablespoon of cookie dough on the coookie sheet.
- Add more dough to make 16 coookies.
- Fluctuate each cookie using your fingers.
- Water for 25 minutes until dawn.
- Let them rest for 15 minutes.
- Serve.

Nutrition: Calories 192 Fat: 17.44g. Carbohydrates: 2.2g. Protein: 4.7g. Fiber: 2.1g.

74) Coconut Cookies

Preparation time: 10 mnutes   **Cooking time:** 20 minutes   **Servings:** 6

Ingredients:
- 6 tablespoons coconut flour
- ¾ teaspoons baking powder
- 1/8 teaspoon sea salt
- 3 tablespoons of nut butter

Directions:
- Preheat our oven to 375 degrees F. Layer a cookie sheet with parchment.
- Place all wet ingredients in a blender. Blend all the mixture in a blender.
- Add the wet mixture and mix well until used up.

Ingredients:
- 1/6 cup coconut oil
- 6 tablespoon data sugar
- 1/3 cup coco nut milk
- 1/2 teaspoon vanilla essence

- Place a spoonful of dough cookie on the cookie sheet.
- Add a little more butter to make many coookies. Bake until golden brown (about 10 minutes). We'll see.

Nutrition: Calories 151 Fat: 13.4g. Carbs: 6.4g. Protein: 4.2g. Fiber: 4.8g

75) Berry Mousse

Preparation time: 5 minutes   **Cooking time:** 5 minutes   **Servings:** 2

Ingredients:
- 1 teaspoon Seville orange zest
- 3 oz. raspberries or blueberries

Directions:
- Blend the rice in an electric blender until the fluff is dissolved.
- Add the vanilla and Seville zest. Stir well.
- Add the walnuts and berries.

Ingredients:
- ¼ teaspoon vanilla essence
- 2 cups coconut cream

- Cover the glove with a plastic wrench.
- Refrigerate for 3 hours.
- Garnish as desired. Serve.

Nutrition: Calories 265 Fat: 13g. Carbohydrates: 7.5g. Protein: 5.2g. Fiber: 0.5g.

76) Coconut pulp Coookies

Preparation time: 5 minutes.   **Cooking time:** 10 hours.   **Servings:** 4

Ingredients:
- 3 cups coconut pulp
- 1 Granny Smith apple
- 1-2 teaspoon cinnamon

Ingredients:
- 2-3 tablespoons of raw honey
- 1/4 cup coco walnut flakes

Directions:
- Blend the coconut with the remaining ingredients in a processor food processor.
- Make many cookies with this mixture.
- Arrange them on a kitchen table, lined with parchment.
- Place the dough in a food grade oven for 6-10 hours at 115 degrees Fahrenheit.
- Serve.

Nutrition: Calories 240 Fat: 22.5g. Carbohydrates: 17.3g. Protein: 14.9g. Fiber: 0g.

77) Avocado Pudding

Preparation time: 10 minutes **Cooking time:** 0 minutes **Servings:** 2

Ingredients:
- 2 avocados
- 3/4-1 cup coconut milk
- 1/3-1/2 cup of raw cacao powder

Ingredients:
- 1 teaspoon 100% pure organic vanilla (optional)
- 2-4 tablespoons of date sugar

Directions:
- Mix all ingredients together in a blender.
- Refrigerate for 4 hours in a container.
- Serve.

Nutrition: Calories 609 Fats: 50.5g. Carbs: 9.9g. Protein: 29.3g. Fiber: 1.5g.

78) Coconut Raisins cooookies

Preparation time: 10 minutes. **Cooking time:** 10 minutes. **Servings:** 4

Ingredients:
- 1 1/4 cups of coconut flour 1 cup of nut flour
- 1 teaspoon baking soda
- 1/2 Celtic teaspoon sea salt
- 1 button for peanuts cup
- 1 cup coconut date sugar

Ingredients:
- 2 teaspoons of vanilla
- ¼ cup coconut milk
- 3/4 cup organic raisins
- 3/4 cup coconut chips or flakes

Directions:
- Turn on the oven to 357 degrees F.
- Mix the flour with the salt and baking soda.
- Flatten with sugar until started and then stirs in the nut milk and vinavilla.
- Mix well, then place in a powder container. Stir until fine.
- Add all remaining ingredients.
- Make small cooookies out this dough.
- Arrange the cookies on a baking sheet.
- Bake for 10 minutes until set.

Nutrition: Calories 237 Fat: 19.8g. Carbs: 55.1g. Protein: 17.8g. Fiber: 0.9g.

79) Cracker Pumpkin Spice

Preparation time: 10 minutes. **Cooking time:** 1 hour. **Servings:** 6

Ingredients:
- 1/3 cup coco walnut flour
- 2 tablespoons pumpkin pie spice
- ¾ cup sunflower seds
- ¾ cup flaxseed
- 1/3 cup sesame seeds

Ingredients:
- 1 tablespoon gron psyllium husk powder
- 1 teaspoon sea salt
- 3 tablespoons coco walnut oil, melted
- 1 1/3 cups water

Directions:
- Heat our oven to 300 degrees F. Combine all ingredients in a bowl.
- Add the salt and oil to the mixture and mix well.
- Allow the dough to rest for 2 to 3 minutes.
- Roll out the dough on a cookie sheet lined with parchment paper.
- Bake for 30 minutes.
- Reduce the amount of food to 30 m weight and let it rest for another 30 m.
- Crush the bread into small pieces. Serve

Nutrition: Calories 248 Fat: 15.7g. Carbs: 0.4g. Protein: 24.9g. Fiber: 0g.

80) Spicy Toasted nuts

Preparation time: 10 minutes. **Cooking time:** 15 minutes. **Servings:** 4

Ingredients:
- 8 ounces of pecans or coconuts or walnuts
- 1 teaspoon of sea salt
- 1 tablespoon olive oil or coconut oil

Ingredients:
- 1 teaspoon of ground cumin
- 1 teaspoon of paprika powder or chili powder

Directions:
- Add all ingredients to an oven. Brown nuts until golden brown.
- Serve and enjoy.

Nutrition: Calories 287 Fat: 29.5g. Carbohydrates: 5.9g. Protein: 4.2g. Fiber: 4.3g.

Chapter 6 -   Dessert Recipes

81) Cracker Healthy

Preparation time: **Cooking time:** 30 minutes **Servings:** 50 Crackers

Ingredients:
- ✓ 1/2 cup of rye flour
- ✓ 1 cup of flour Spelt
- ✓ 2 teaspoons of Sesame Seed
- ✓ 1 teaspoon of Agave Syrup

Directions:
- ❖ Preheat our oven to 350 degrees Fahrenheit.
- ❖ Add all ingredients to a glass container and mix everything together.
- ❖ Make a ball of dough. If the dough is too thick, add more flour.
- ❖ Prepare a place to spread the dough and cover it with a piece of parchment paper.
- ❖ Degrease the container well with Grape Seed Oil and put the dart in it.
- ❖ RICE the slurry with a rolling pin, adding more flour so it doesn't fall apart.

Ingredients:
- ✓ 1 teaspoon of Pure Sea Salt
- ✓ 2 tablespoons of Grape Seed Oil
- ✓ 3/4 cup of Spring Water

- ❖ When your dough is ready, take a pastry cutter and insert it into the container. If you don't have a pastry cutter, you can use a cookie cutter.
- ❖ Arrange the squares on a kitchen basket and place them in the corner of a ech square using a fork of a skewer.
- ❖ Brush the plate with a little grain oil and sprinkle with a little pure sea salt, if needed.
- ❖ Bake for 12-15 minutes or until crackers are golden brown.
- ❖ Everything that was done was done with the help of another person.
- ❖ Serve and enjoy your Healthy Crackers!

Nutrition: Calories

Helpful Hints: You can add any seasonings from the Doctor Sebi's food list according to your desire. You can make crackers with our tomato sauce, avocado sauce or cheese. Sauce.

82) Tortillas

Preparation time:. **Cooking Time:** 20 Minutes **Servings:** 8

Ingredients:
- ✓ 2 cups of flour Spelt
- ✓ 1 teaspoon of Pure Sea Salt

Directions:
- ❖ In a food processor* blend the spelt flour with the pure salt. Blend for about 15 minutes.
- ❖ Blend, slowly add Grape seed oil until well distributed.
- ❖ Slowly add the soy water, stirring until a color forms.
- ❖ Prepare a piece of wallpaper and pour some parchment paper on it. Dust with a little flour.

Ingredients:
- ✓ 1/2 cup of spring Water

- ❖ Process the nut for about 1 to 2 minutes until it reaches the right consistency.
- ❖ Pour dough into 8-inch pieces.
- ❖ Roll the sandwich into a very thin shape.
- ❖ Prepare a lunch box, cook one tortilla at a time in the microwave for about 30-60 minutes.
- ❖ Serve and enjoy your Tortillas!

Nutrition: Calories

Helpful Hints: If you don't have a refrigerator, you can use a mixer or blender. However, you will have a better result with a food as you have nothing to do with. You can serve the Tortillas with our Sweet Butter Sauce, Avocado Sauce or Cheese. Sauce.

83) Walnut cheesecake Mango

Preparation time: **Cooking time:** 4 hours and 30 minutes **Servings:** 8

Ingredients:
- ✓ 2 cups of Brazil Nuts
- ✓ 5 to 6 Dates
- ✓ 1 tablespoon of Sea Moss Gel (check information)
- ✓ 1/4 cup o of agave syrup
- ✓ 1/4 teaspoon salt Pure Sea
- ✓ 2 tablespoons of Lime Juice
- ✓ 1 1/2 cups of Homemade Walnut Milk *

Directions:
- ❖ Place all crust ingredients in a processor and blend for 30 seconds.
- ❖ Prepare a baking sheet with a sheet of parchment and roll out the loose dough with butter.
- ❖ Place the Mango sliced across the crust and freeze for 10 minutes.
- ❖ Place all the glass pieces in a bowl until ready.

Ingredients:
Crust:
- ✓ 1 1/2 cups of quartered Dates 1/4 cup of Agave Syrup
- ✓ 1 1/2 cups of Coconut Flakes
- ✓ 1/4 teaspoon of Pure Sea Salt
- ✓ Toppings:
- ✓ Mango of Sliced
- ✓ Sliced strawberries
- ❖ Place the filling on top of the butter, wrap it with aluminum foil or a food container and let it rest for 3 to 4 hours in the refrigerator.
- ❖ Take out dalla baking form and garnish with toppings.
- ❖ Serve and enjoy our Mango Nut Cheesecake!

Nutrition: Calories

Helpful Hints: If you don't have homemade nut milk, you can use Homemade hemp seed milk.

84) Blackberry Jam

Preparation time: **Cooking time:** 4 hours and 30 minutes **Servings:** 1 cup

Ingredients:
- 3/4 cup of Blackberries
- 1 tablespoon lime juice Key

Ingredients:
- 3 tablespoons of Agave Syrup
- ¼ cup of Sea Moss Gel + extra 2 tablespoons (check information)

Directions:
- Place blackberries in a medium saucepan and cook over low heat.
- Stir in blackberries until liquid is gone.
- Once you've picked the berries, use your blender to chop up the larger pieces. If you don't have a blender, put the mixture in an immersion blender, blend it well, and then return it to the oven.
- Add Sea Moss Gel, Key Lime Juice and Agave Syrup to the mixture. Cook over low heat and stir well until dry.
- Remove from heat and let sit for 10 minutes.
- Serve with pieces on flat bread.
- Enjoy your jam!

Nutrition: Calories

Helpful Hints: If you don't have Sea Moss Gel, you can omit it. However, the gel gives your skin a thinner, longer-lasting look. Blackberries have a natural pectin, which can have a similar effect. Store this Blackberry Jam in a glass jar with a lid in the refrigerator for 2 to 3 weeks. Do not store in extreme temperatures!

85) Blackberry Bars

Preparation time: **Cooking time:** 1 hour 20 Minutes **Servings:** 4

Ingredients:
- 3 Burro Banas or 4 Baby Banas
- 1 cup of Spelt Flour
- 2 cups of Quinoa Flakes
- 1/4 cup of Agave Syrup

Ingredients:
- 1/4 teaspoon of Pure Sea Salt
- 1/2 cup of Grape Seed Oil
- 1 cup of prepared Blackberry Jam

Directions:
- Set the oven to 350 degrees Fahrenheit.
- Mash the bananas with a fork in a large bowl.
- Combine Agave Syrup and Grape Seed Oil to the puree and mix well.
- Add the Spelt flour and Quinoa flakes. Knead the dough until it becomes sticky to your finger.
- Prepare a 9x9-inch basket with a parchment lid.
- Take 2/3 of the dough and spread it with your fingers on the baking sheet parchment pan.
- Spread Blackberry Jam over the dough.
- Crumble the rice and place it on the plate.
- Bake for 20 minutes.
- Remove from oven and let cool for 10-15 minutes.
- Cut into small pieces.
- Try and enjoy our Blackberry Bars!

Nutrition: Calories

Helpful Hints: You can store this Blackberry Bar in the refrigerator for 5-6 days or in the freezer for up to 3 months.

86) Squash Pie.

Preparation time: **Cooking time:** 2 hours 30 Minutes **Servings:** 6-8

Ingredients:
- 2 Butternut Squashes
- 1 1/4 cups of spelt flour
- 1/4 cup of dry sugar
- 1/4 cup of Agave Syrup
- 1 teaspoon of Allspice.

Ingredients:
- 1 teaspoon of Pure Sea Salt
- 1/4 cup soy water
- 1/3 cup of fat seed oil
- 1/4 cup hemp seed milk Homemade *

Directions:
- Rinse and peel butternut pumpkins.
- Cut them in half and use a spoon to de-sed.
- Cut the meat into one piece and place in a glass container.
- Cover the squash in Spring Water and boiltare for 20-25 minutes until coooked.
- Turn off the oven and mash the cooked squash.
- Add the date sugar, agave syrup, 1/8 pure sea salt, and homemade milk and mix everything together.
- Crust:
- Preheat the oven to 350 degrees Fahrenheit.
- In a bowl, add the spelt flour, 1/2 teaspoon of Pure Sea Salt, Spring Water, and Grape Seed Oil and mix.
- Reduce the rice into a loaf of bread. Add more water or flour if needed. Let stand for 5 minutes.
- Spread out Spelt Flour on a piece of parchment paper.
- Roll out on rolling pin, adding more flour to prevent sticking.
- Place the dough in a cake pan and bake for 10 minutes.
- Remove the butter from the oven, add the filling and bake for another 40 minutes.
- Remove the cake and let it rest for 30 minutes until cool.
- Serve enjoy your Squash Pie!

Nutrition: Calories

Helpful Hints:

87) Walnut Milk homemade

Preparation time: **Cooking time:** minimum 8 hours **Servings:** 4 cups

Ingredients:
- ✓ 1 cup fresh walnuts
- ✓ 1/8 teaspoon of Pure Sea Salt

Ingredients:
- ✓ 3 cups of spring water + extra for soaking

Directions:
- ❖ Place the new Walnuts in a bag and fill it with three tablespoons of water.
- ❖ Take the Walnuts for an hour and a half.
- ❖ Drain and rinse nuts with warm water.
- ❖ Add the soaked walnuts, puree and three times the spring water to a blender.
- ❖ Mix well till smooth.
- ❖ Extend it if you need to.
- ❖ Enjoy your homemade nut milk!

Nutrition: Calories

Helpful Hints:

88) Aquafaba

Preparation time: **Cooking time:** 2 Hours 30 minutes **Servings:** 2-4 cups

Ingredients:
- ✓ 1 bag of Garbanzo beans
- ✓ 1 teaspoon of Pure Sea Salt

Ingredients:
- ✓ 6 cups of Spring Water + extra for soaking

Directions:
- ❖ Place the chickpeas in a large pot, add the soy water and pure sea salt. Bring to a boil.
- ❖ Remove from heat and allow to soak 30 to 40 minutes.
- ❖ Strain the Garbanzo Beans and add 6 cups of water.
- ❖ Boil for 1 hour and 30 minutes on medium hat.
- ❖ Filter the Garbanzo beans. This filtered water is Aquafaba.
- ❖ Pour the Aquafaba into a glass jar with a lid and place in the refrigerator.
- ❖ After cooling, the Aquafaba becomes thicker. If it is too thick, boil for 10-20 mnutes.

Nutrition: Calories

Helpful hints: Aquafaba is a good alternative for one egg: 2 tablespoons of Aquafaba = 1 egg white; 3 tablespoons of Aquafaba = 1 egg.

89) Milk Homemade Hempsed

Preparation time: **Cooking time:** 2 hours   **Servings:** 2 cups

Ingredients:
- 2 tablespoons of Hemp Seeds
- 2 tablespoons of Agave Syrup

Ingredients:
- 1/8 teaspoon pure salt
- 2 cups of Spring Water Fruits (optional)*.

Directions:
- Place all ingredients, except fruit, in blender.
- Blend them for two minutes.
- Add fruits and resin for 30-50 minutes.

- Store milk in the refrigerator until aged.
- Enjoy your Homemade Hempsed Milk!

Nutrition: Calories

Helpful Hints:

90) Oil spicy infusion

Preparation time: **Cooking time:** 24 Hours   **Servings:** 1 cup

Ingredients:
- 1 tablespoon of crushed Cayenne Pepper

Ingredients:
- 3/4 cup of Grape Seed Oil

Directions:
- Fill a glass with a lid or bottle with grape oil.
- Add crushed Cayenne Pepper to the jar/bottle.

- Close and allow to cool for at least 24 hours.
- Add it to a dinner party and enjoy our Spicy Infuse oil!

Nutrition: Calories

Helpful Hints:

91) Italian infused oil

Preparation time: **Cooking time:** 24 hours   **Servings:** 1 cup

Ingredients:
- 1 teaspoon of Oregano.
- 1 teaspoon of Basil

Ingredients:
- 1 pinch of salt Pure Sea
- 3/4 cup of Grape seed oil

Directions:
- Fill a glass jar with a lid or container with grape oil.
- Mix the seasonings and add them to the rice and lettuce.

- Shake and let the oil steep for at least 24 hours.
- Add it to a dish and enjoy your Infused Oil Italian!

Nutrition: Calories

Helpful Hints:

92) Garlic Infused Oil

Preparation time: **Cooking time:** 24 hours   **Servings:** 1 cup

Ingredients:
- 1/2 teaspoon of Dill
- 1/2 teaspoon of Ginger Powder
- 1 tablespoon of Onion Powder.

Ingredients:
- 1/2 teaspoon of Pure Sea Salt
- 3/4 cup of fat seed oil

Directions:
- Fill a glass jar or squeeze bottle with grapeseed oil.
- Add the seasonings to the jar/bottle.

- Close and let oil infuse for at least 24 hours.
- Add it to a dish and add your "Garlic". Infused Oil!

Nutrition: Calories

Helpful Hints:

93) Papaya Seeds Mango Dressing

Preparation time: **Cooking time**: 10 minutes **Servings**: 1/2 Cup

Ingredients:
- ✓ 1 cup of chopped Mango
- ✓ 1 teaspoon of Papaya Seeds Ground
- ✓ 1 teaspoon of Basil
- ✓ 1 teaspoon of Onion Powder

Directions:
- ❖ Prepare and place all ingredients into the mixture.
- ❖ Blend for one minute until smoth.

Nutrition: Calories

Helpful Hints:

Ingredients:
- ✓ 1 teaspoon of Agave Syrup
- ✓ 2 tablespoons of lemon juice
- ✓ 1/4 cup of grape oil
- ✓ 1/4 teaspoon salt Pure Sea
- ❖ Add it to a dish and enjoy our Papaya Seed Mango Dress5ng!

94) Blueberry Smoothie

Preparation time: 10 minutes **Cooking time**: **Servings**: 2

Ingredients:
- ✓ 2 cups of frozen blueberries
- ✓ 1 small banana

Directions:
- ❖ Place all ingredients in a high speed blender and pulse until creamy.

Nutrition: Calories

Helpful Hints:

Ingredients:
- ✓ 1½ cups unsweetened almond milk
- ✓ ¼ cup ice cubes
- ❖ Pour the smoothie into two glasses and serve immediately.

95) Raspberry and tofu smoothie

Preparation time: 10 minutes **Cooking time**: **Servings**: 2

Ingredients:
- ✓ 1½ cups of fresh raspberries
- ✓ 6 ounces of firm silken tofu, pressed and drained
- ✓ 4-5 drops of liquid stevia

Directions:
- ❖ Place all ingredients in a high speed blender and pulse until creamy.

Nutrition: Calories

Helpful Hints:

Ingredients:
- ✓ 1 cup of coconut cream
- ✓ ¼ cup ice, crushed
- ❖ Pour the smoothie into two glasses and serve immediately.

96) Beet and Strawberry Smoothie

Preparation time: 10 minutes **Cooking time**: **Servings**: 2

Ingredients:
- ✓ 2 cups frozen strawberries, pitted and chopped
- ✓ ⅔ cup roasted and frozen beet, chopped
- ✓ 1 teaspoon fresh ginger, peeled and grated

Directions:
- ❖ Place all ingredients in a high speed blender and pulse until creamy.

Nutrition: Calories

Helpful Hints:

Ingredients:
- ✓ 1 teaspoon fresh turmeric, peeled and grated
- ✓ ½ cup of fresh orange juice
- ✓ 1 cup unsweetened almond milk
- ❖ Pour the smoothie into two glasses and serve immediately.

97) Kiwi Smoothie

Preparation time: 10 minutes   **Cooking time**:   **Servings**: 2

Ingredients:
- 4 kiwis
- 2 small bananas, peeled
- 1½ cups unsweetened almond milk
- 1-2 drops of liquid stevia
- ¼ cup ice cubes

Directions:
- Place all ingredients in a high speed blender and pulse until creamy.
- Pour the smoothie into two glasses and serve immediately.

Nutrition: Calories

Helpful Hints:

98) Pineapple and Carrot Smoothie

Preparation time: 10 minutes   **Cooking time**:   **Servings**: 2

Ingredients:
- 1 cup frozen pineapple
- 1 large ripe banana, peeled and sliced
- ½ tablespoon fresh ginger, peeled and chopped
- ¼ teaspoon ground turmeric
- 1 cup unsweetened almond milk
- ½ cup fresh carrot juice
- 1 tablespoon fresh lemon juice

Directions:
- Place all ingredients in a high speed blender and pulse until creamy.
- Pour the smoothie into two glasses and serve immediately.

Nutrition: Calories

Helpful Hints:

99) Oatmeal and orange smoothie

Preparation time: 10 minutes   **Cooking time**:   **Servings**: 4

Ingredients:
- ⅔ cup of rolled oats
- 2 oranges, peeled, seeds removed and cut into sections
- 2 large bananas, peeled and sliced
- 2 cups of unsweetened almond milk
- 1 cup ice cubes, crushed

Directions:
- Place all ingredients in a high speed blender and pulse until creamy.
- Pour the smoothie into four glasses and serve immediately.

Nutrition: Calories

Helpful Hints:

100) Pumpkin Smoothie

Preparation time: 10 minutes   **Cooking time**:   **Servings**: 2

Ingredients:
- 1 cup homemade pumpkin puree
- 1 medium banana, peeled and sliced
- 1 tablespoon maple syrup
- 1 teaspoon ground flax seeds
- ½ teaspoon ground cinnamon
- ¼ teaspoon ground ginger
- 1½ cups unsweetened almond milk
- ¼ cup ice cubes

Directions:
- Place all ingredients in a high speed blender and pulse until creamy.
- Pour the smoothie into two glasses and serve immediately.

Nutrition: Calories

Chapter 7 - Dr. Lewis's Meal Plan Project

Day 1

1) Blueberry Muffins
23) Vegetable and berry salad
41) Mixed stew of spicy vegetables
64) Mediterranean peppers
86) Squash Pie.

Day 2

4) "Chocolate" Pudding.
25) Grab and Go Wraps
46) Curried red beans
61) Quinoa Salad
100) Pumpkin Smoothie

Day 3

7) Strawberry and Beet Smoothie
28) Avocado and salmon soup
51) Quinoa with vegetables
67) Alkalized vegetable lasagna
87) Walnut Milk homemade

Day 4

11) Orange and Oat Smoothie
31) Spicy cabbage bowl
55) Chickpeas with pumpkin
73) Coconut cookies Chip
99) Oatmeal and orange smoothie

Day 5

18) Pecan Pancakes
33) Vegan Burger
58) Green beans and mushrooms in casserole
71) Homemade Protein Bar
82) Tortillas

Day 6

16) Hemp seed and carrot muffins
37) Walnut, date, orange and cabbage salad
59) Meatloaf of wild rice and lentils
80) Spicy Toasted nuts
89) Milk Homemade Hempsed

Day 7

19) Quinoa Breakfast
40) Alkalizing millet dish
54) Spicy baked beans
77) Avocado Pudding
83) Walnut cheesecake Mango

Chapter 8 - Conclusion

I hope this book can lead you to your goals, keeping your desire to keep going high, without making you lose sight of the outcome

This book series is designed to help women, men, athletes and sportsmen, people immersed in work with little free time, etc.

If you recognize yourself in one of these categories or someone you know has decided to take the same path as you,

You'll find the other books in the series in your trusted bookstore, guaranteed!

Big hugs from Dr. Grace!

Alkaline Diet Cookbook for Athletes

Dr. Lewis's Meal Plan Project| How to Boost Sports Performance by Balancing Body Acids Without Giving Up Your Favorite Foods| 100 Energetic Recipes to Take Your Favorite Sport to The Highest Level

By Grace Lewis

Chapter 1 - Introduction

Are you looking for an effective path that can take your sports performance to the next level?

The alkaline diet is for you!

Here are some of the main benefits claimed by proponents of the alkaline diet, and the scientific research to back them up:

- *Prevention of osteoporosis*
- *Promoting weight loss*
- *Preventing cancer*
- *Treating or preventing heart disease*
- *Improving back pain*
- *Improving kidney health*
- *Improving growth hormone levels*

The important thing to remember about nutrition is that it usually requires self-sacrifice and discipline. After a hard day of training, it is vital to replenish your body daily by preparing essential foods. This is where supplements come in. Supplements offer a convenient alternative to a non-traditional diet.

When following an alkaline diet, it is essential to find a supplement that fits the diet and promotes an alkaline environment in the body. Dietary supplementation contains plant extracts, essential fatty acids, food extracts and high fibre content.

By incorporating an alkaline diet into their nutritional regime, most athletes notice an improvement in endurance, energy levels and stamina. Some athletes also undergo a mild cleansing process as some lose body fat, improve their well-being and strengthen their immune system. By fine-tuning your diet as much as possible, you can take your athleticism to another level.

At the end of this book you will find my personal diet plan suitable for athletes, able to make you experience right away the enormous benefits that the alkaline diet can offer.

Enjoy your meal!

Grace

Chapter 2 -   Breakfast Recipes

1) Baked Grapefruit

Preparation time: **Cooking time:**   **Servings:** 1

Ingredients:
- *Unsweetened grated coconut, 2 tablespoons*
- Halved grapefruit, 1

Directions:
- You will need to heat the oven to 350.
- Take some foil and line a baking sheet with it.
- Place grapefruits cut in half with cut side up on aluminum foil. Cover each with a tablespoon of coconut.
- Place in oven and bake 15 minutes or until coconut is tan.
- Carefully remove from oven and enjoy.

2) Almond Fritters

Preparation time: **Cooking time:**   **Servings:** 4

Ingredients:
- Coconut oil, 3 tablespoons
- Almond milk, 1 c.
- Baking powder, 1 teaspoon
- Arrowroot powder, 2 tablespoons
- Almond flour, 1 c.

Directions:
- Place each of the dry fixings in a dish and whisk to mix.
- Add two tablespoons of coconut oil along with the almond milk to the dry items and mix well until everything is blended.
- Place a skillet over medium heat and put a teaspoon of coconut in to melt. Swirl it around in the pan to coat it.
- Pour a ladleful of batter into the pan and use the bottom of the ladle to smooth the pancake.
- Bake for three minutes until the edges are bubbly and brown.
- Flip the pancake over and bake another three minutes until cooked through.
- Continue to cook the pancakes until all the batter has been used.

3) Amaranth Porridge

Preparation time: **Cooking time:**   **Servings:** 2

Ingredients:
- Cinnamon, 1 tablespoon
- Coconut oil, 2 tablespoons
- Amaranth, 1 c.
- Alkaline water, 2 c.
- Almond milk, 2 c.

Directions:
- Place the water and milk in a pot. Set to medium-hot and allow to boil.
- Add the amaranth and lower the heat to low. Stew for half an hour, stirring occasionally.
- Remove from heat, add copra oil and cinnamon, mix well, serve hot.

4) Banana Porridge

Preparation time: **Cooking time:**   **Servings:** 2

Ingredients:
- Chopped almonds, .25 c.
- Liquid stevia, 3 drops
- Barley, .5 c.
- Sliced banana, 1
- Unsweetened almond milk, 1 c.

Directions:
- Mix stevia, 1/2 cup almond milk and barley in a bowl.
- Refrigerate, covered for six hours.
- Remove from refrigerator and stir in remaining milk. Pour into a saucepan and place on medium. Allow mixture to cook for five minutes.

5) Zucchini Muffins

Preparation time: **Cooking time:** **Servings: 16**

Ingredients:
- Halls
- Cinnamon, 1 teaspoon
- Baking powder, 1 tablespoon
- Almond flour, 2 c.
- Vanilla extract, 1 teaspoon
- Almond milk, .5 c.
- Grated zucchini, 2

Ingredients:
- Overripe bananas, 3
- Almond butter, .25 c.
- Alkaline water, 3 tablespoons
- Ground flaxseed, 1 tablespoon
- Optional Ingredients:
- Chopped walnuts, .25 c.
- Chocolate chips, .25 c.

Directions:
- You need to heat your cooking appliance to 375 degrees. Spray a cupcake pan with cooking spray.
- Place the water and flaxseed in a bowl.
- Mash the bananas in a pot and put all the leftover contents in. Stir well.
- Separate the concoction evenly into a cupcake pan.
- Place in oven for 25 minutes.

6) Tofu Stew With Vegetables

Preparation time: **Cooking time:** **Servings: 4**

Ingredients:
- Halls
- Chopped basil, 2 tablespoons
- Chopped firm tofu, 3 c.
- Diced peppers (red, bell), 2 pieces.
- Olive oil, 1 tablespoon

Ingredients:
- Turmeric
- Chopped cherry tomatoes, 2 c.
- Chopped onions, 2
- Cayenne

Directions:
- Place a greased skillet over medium heat and heat the pan.
- Place peppers along with onions, prepare for five minutes.
- Add the tofu, cayenne, salt and turmeric. Cook an additional eight minutes.
- Garnish with the basil.

7) Zucchini Fritters

Preparation time: **Cooking time:** **Servings: 8**

Ingredients:
- Finely chopped shallots, .5 c.
- Jalapeno finely chopped, 2
- Olive oil, 2 tablespoons
- Ground flaxseed, 4 tablespoons

Ingredients:
- Halls
- Grated zucchini, 6
- Alkaline water, 12 tablespoons

Directions:
- Place flaxseed and water in a bowl and mix well. Set aside.
- Place a large skillet over medium heat and heat the oil. Add the pepper, salt and zucchini. Cook three minutes and place zucchini in a bowl.
- Add the flaxseed mixture and scallions and mix well.
- Heat a griddle that has been sprayed with cooking spray. Pour some zucchini onto the preheated griddle and cook three minutes per side until golden brown.
- Repeat until the mixture is completely used up.

8) Pumpkin Quinoa

Preparation time: **Cooking time:** **Servings: 2**

Ingredients:
- Chia seeds, 2 teaspoons
- Pumpkin pie spice, 1 teaspoon
- Pumpkin puree, .25 c.

Ingredients:
- Crushed banana, 1
- Unsweetened almond milk, 1 c.
- Cooked quinoa, 1 c.

Directions:
- Place all ingredients in a container.
- Make sure the lid is sealed and shake well to combine.
- Refrigerate overnight.
- When it's ready to eat, take it out of the fridge and enjoy.

9) Avocado Toast

Preparation time: **Cooking time:** **Servings: 4**

Ingredients:
- ✓ Dulse flakes, sliced radish, sliced red onion, for garnish - optional
- ✓ Sea salt, 0.5 teaspoons
- ✓ Fresh coriander leaves, 1 tablespoon
- ✓ Chopped onion, 1 tablespoon

Ingredients:
- ✓ Garlic, 2 cloves
- ✓ Jalapeno
- ✓ Avocado, 2
- ✓ Sweet potato, unpeeled, cut into 4 thick slices lengthwise

Directions:
- ❖ Place each of the potato slices in a slot of the toaster oven and toast them for four cycles, or until they are cooked through. You can also toast them in the oven if you don't have a regular toaster oven. You want them to be tender enough that you can easily pierce them with a fork. Carefully arrange the cooked "toasts" on plates.
- ❖ While the sweet potato toast is cooking, add the salt, cilantro, onion, garlic, jalapeno and avocado to an extremely electric food processor and blend until smooth. Adjust the amount of salt as needed.
- ❖ Divide the avocado spread over each of the sweet potato toast slices. Top each slice with desired toppings. Enjoy.

10) Frozen Banana Breakfast Bowl

Preparation time: **Cooking time:** **Servings: 1**

Ingredients:
- ✓ Chia seeds, hemp seeds, unsweetened coconut flakes, for garnish - optional
- ✓ Pumpkin seed protein powder, 4 tablespoons

Ingredients:
- ✓ Bananas, 2

Directions:
- ❖ Peel and then slice the bananas. Place them thinly in a freezer safe container and freeze overnight.
- ❖ The next morning, add the bananas to a food processor and blend until you reach a creamy, smooth consistency, much like soft-serve ice cream.
- ❖ Process the pumpkin protein powder through the bananas until just combined.
- ❖ Pour into a serving dish and add desired toppings, if desired, and enjoy.

11) Cobbler Of Chia Seeds And Blueberries

Preparation time: **Cooking time:** **Servings: 4**

Ingredients:
- ✓ Blueberry Blend -
- ✓ Chia seeds, 1 tablespoon
- ✓ Unrefined whole cane sugar, 2 tablespoons
- ✓ Blueberries, 2 c.
- ✓ Topping -
- ✓ Almond flour, .5 c.
- ✓ Sea salt, .25 teaspoon
- ✓ Vanilla bean powder, 1 teaspoon

Ingredients:
- ✓ A mixture of baking soda and cream of tartar, 1.5 teaspoons
- ✓ Unrefined whole cane sugar, 2 tablespoons
- ✓ Melted coconut oil, 2 tablespoons
- ✓ Coconut milk, 4 tablespoons
- ✓ Oatmeal, .5 c.

Directions:
- ❖ Start by setting your oven to 350.
- ❖ To make the blueberries, mix the chia seeds, sugar and blueberries. Place blueberry mixture in the bottom of four 4-ounce baking cups.
- ❖ To fix the topping, mix together the salt, vanilla powder, baking powder, sugar, coconut oil, coconut milk, oatmeal and almond flour.
- ❖ Divide the blueberry topping among the four ramekins. You can leave the topping by spoonfuls, or you can spread it evenly over the blueberry mixture to create a complete crust.
- ❖ Bake the cobblers for 45 minutes, or until the topping has turned golden brown and everything is heated through. Enjoy.

12) Quick And Easy Granola Bars

Preparation time: 10 Minutes   **Cooking time:** 15-20 Minutes   **Servings:** 6

Ingredients:
- Vanilla bean powder, .25 teaspoon
- Cinnamon spice, .25 teaspoon
- Sea salt, .25 teaspoon
- Coconut oil, 1 tablespoon

Directions:
- Place some parchment in the bottom of a 9x5 inch baking dish.
- Add the vanilla bean powder, cinnamon, salt, coconut oil, brown rice syrup, almond butter and oats to a food processor and blend until well combined.

Ingredients:
- Brown rice syrup, 2 tablespoons
- Almond butter, .5 c.
- Quick rolled oats, 1 c.

- Slide the dough into the pan and push it down into an even dough, making sure it's firmly compressed. Refrigerate the bars for 15-20 minutes, or until they are completely firm.
- Cut granola into six bars and enjoy. Store leftovers in the refrigerator. At room temperature, they will become soft.

13) Alkaline Blueberry Spelt Pancakes

Preparation time: 6 mnutes.   **Cooking time:** 20 minutes.   **Servings:** 3

Ingredients:
- 2 cups of spelt flour
- 1 cup coconut Milk
- 1/2 cup Alkaline Water
- 2 tbsps. Grape sed Oil

Directions:
- Mix together in a whisk the flower spellate, agave, wheat sed oil, hemp seeds and moss5s together.
- To the menstruum, add 1 cup of sheep's milk and cologne until you get the consistency menstruum you like.

Ingredients:
- 1/2 cup Agave
- 1/2 cup Blueberries
- 1/4 teaspoon of musk Sea

- Mash the blue into the batter.
- Heat over medium heat and then lightly coat with the cereal oil.
- Place the butter in the oven and let it cook for about 5 minutes on all sides.
- Serve and have fun.

14) Blueberry Alkaline Muffins

Preparation time: 5 Minutes.   **Cooking time:** 20 minutes.   **Servings:** 3

Ingredients:
- 1 cup of coconut milk
- 3/4 cup of Spelt Flour
- 3/4 Teff of flour
- 1/2 cup Blueberries

Directions:
- Adjust the oven temperature to 365 degrees.
- Grate 6 regular-size muffin cups with muffin liners.
- In a bowl, mix the sea salt, moss, agave, nut milk and flour until liquid.

Ingredients:
- 1/3 cup of Agave
- 1/4 cup Sea Moss Gel
- 1/2 teaspoon coarse salt, ground salt, olive oil

- Then crimp in blueberries.
- Lightly cover the muffins with the wheat seeds.
- Pour in the batter of muffin.
- Bake for at least 30 minutes until golden brown.
- Serve.

15) Meal Of Crispy Quinoa

Preparation time: 5 minutes **Cooking time:** 25 minutes. **Servings: 2**

Ingredients:
- ✓ 3 cups of nut milk coco
- ✓ 1 cup rinsed quinoa.
- ✓ 1/8 tsp. cinnamon powder

Directions:
- ❖ In a saucepan, your milk and bring to a boil over moderate heat.
- ❖ Add the milk to the milk and then bring it to soak once more.
- ❖ Then let sit for at least 15 minutes over medium heat until the milk has reduced.

Ingredients:
- ✓ 1 cup raspberry
- ✓ 1/2 coconut

- ❖ Stand higher in the corner than in the middle of the world.
- ❖ Cook for 8 minutes until milk is ready to use.
- ❖ Add the raspberry and coook the meal for 30 seconds.
- ❖ Serve enjoy.

16) Coconut Pancakes

Preparation time: 5 minutes. **Cooking time:** 15 minutes. **Servings: 4**

Ingredients:
- ✓ 1 cup coconut flour
- ✓ 2 tbsps. Arrow root powder
- ✓ 1 tsp. baking powder

Directions:
- ❖ In a medium container, mix all ingredients together.
- ❖ Add the coconut milk and 2 tbsps. Del coconut oil and mix properly.
- ❖ In a skillet, melt 1 tsp. of coco walnut oil.
- ❖ Pour a ladleful of batter inside the container and then spread the batter evenly on a smooth surface.

Ingredients:
- ✓ 1 cup coco walnut milk
- ✓ 3 tbsps. Coconut oil

- ❖ Coook il form for a least 3 minutes on average heat until you becomes firm.
- ❖ Flip the pancake over to the other side and bake for another 2 minutes until golden brown.
- ❖ Cook the pancakes in a microwave oven.
- ❖ Serve.

17) Quinoa Porridge

Preparation time: 5 minutes. **Cooking time:** 25 minutes. **Servings: 2**

Ingredients:
- ✓ 2 cups coco nut milk
- ✓ 1 cup rinsed quinoa.

Directions:
- ❖ In a saucepan, boil the nut milk at a high temperature.
- ❖ Add the quinoa to the milk and then bring the mixture to a boil.
- ❖ Then you let it sit for 15 mnutes on medium heat until the milk has reduced.

Ingredients:
- ✓ 1/8 tsp. ground cinnamon
- ✓ 1 cup fresh blueberries

- ❖ Add the cinnamon and then mix well in the refrigerator.
- ❖ Bake for at least 8 minutes until the milk is absorbed.
- ❖ Add the blue and light blue and then mix for another 30 seconds.
- ❖ Serve.

18) Amaranth Porridge

Preparation time: 5 minutes. **Cooking time:** 30 minutes. **Servings: 2**

Ingredients:
- ✓ 2 cups coconut milk
- ✓ 2 cups alkaline water
- ✓ 1 cup of administrator

Directions:
- ❖ In a bowl, mix the milk with the water and then boil the milk.

Ingredients:
- ✓ 2 tbsps. Coconut oil
- ✓ 1 tbsp. land cinnamon

- ❖ You put in the amaranth and then reduce the heat and make the milk.

19) Banana Barley Porridge

Preparation time: 15 minutes.   **Cooking time**: 5 minutes.   **Servings**: 2

Ingredients:
- 1 glass divided unsweetened coconut milk
- 1 small bernard cut into slices
- 1/2 cup barley

Directions:
- In a bowl, properly mix barley with half the coconut milk and stevia.
- Cover the bowl and let sit for about 6 hours.

Ingredients:
- 3 drops liquid stevia.
- 1/4 cup chopped coconuts

- In a saucepan, mix the barley mixture with the coconut milk.
- Coook for about 5 minutes on moderate hat.
- Then top with chopped walnuts and bernard.
- Serve.

20) Zucchini Muffins

Preparation time: 10 minutes.   **Cooking time**: 25 minutes.   **Servings**: 16

Ingredients:
- 1 tbsp. ground flaxsed
- 3 tbsps. Alkaline water
- 1/4 inch walnut
- 3 medium over-ripe banas
- 2 small grated zucchinis

Directions:
- Adjust the temperature of your oven to 375°F.
- Grill the muffler tray with the appropriate cover.
- In a bowl, mix the flaxsed with the water.

Ingredients:
- 1/2 cup coco walnut milk
- 1 tsp. vanilla extract
- 2 cups coconut flour
- 1 tbsp. baking powder
- 1 teaspoon of cinnamon 1/4 teaspoon of sea salt

- In a glass tumbler, massh the bananas and remaining ingredients.
- Mix thoroughly and then divide the mixture into the muffin molds.
- Bake for 25 minutes.
- Serve.

Chapter 3 -   Lunch Recipes

21) Green Noodle Salad

Preparation time: **Cooking time:** **Servings: 2**

Ingredients:
- 1 pinch of sea salt
- 1 cup chopped fresh basil
- 2 tablespoons lemon juice, fresh
- ¼ cup unleavened vegetable broth

Directions:
- First, cook the noodles according to package directions. Once ready, drain and rinse under cold running water. Once done, set aside and allow to cool.
- Thinly slice the zucchini and shred the kale. Steam the two vegetables very lightly for a few minutes until the color pops. Make sure they still remain crispy.

Ingredients:
- 1" ginger knob
- 1 cup of kale
- 1 cup zucchini, chopped
- 1 handful of lettuce
- 1 cup millet noodles
- Wash and cut the lettuce and discard the stalks.
- Start by making the dressing: combine the vegetable broth and lemon juice in a food processor, and then add the chopped ginger. Blend the ingredients for about 15-30 seconds.
- Now mix the basil, shredded lettuce, zucchini, cabbage and noodles in a bowl and pour the dressing over it. Mix well and then season with salt.
- Serve and enjoy.

22) Pumpkin Ratatouille

Preparation time: **Cooking time:** **Servings: 4**

Ingredients:
- 1 cup of spring water
- Pinch of cayenne pepper
- Sea salt or organic salt
- 4 tablespoons of cold-pressed extra virgin olive oil
- 2 teaspoons of thyme
- 1 fennel bulb

Directions:
- Cut the bell bell pepper, tomatoes and fresh squash into small portions. Then dice the fennel and onions.
- In a pot, heat some olive oil and then sauté the fennel and onions for a few minutes.

Ingredients:
- 2 large onions
- 1 cup cherry tomatoes, chopped
- 1 red bell pepper
- 1 yellow bell pepper
- 16 ounces of fresh pumpkin

- Now add the bell bell pepper and the squash. Then sauté the mixture for about 8 minutes.
- Once done, add the alkaline water, thyme and tomatoes and cook until the vegetables are quite tender but not too soft.

23) Roasted Vegetables

Preparation time: **Cooking time:** **Servings: 2**

Ingredients:
- A sprinkling of cayenne pepper
- A drizzle of olive oil
- 2 fennel bulbs, chopped
- 1/2 onion, sliced

Directions:
- Preheat the oven to 450 degrees F.
- Then, on a pitted baking sheet, place the fennel bulbs and vegetables and then drizzle everything with a little olive oil.

Ingredients:
- 1 yellow pumpkin, cut into slices
- 1 zucchini, sliced
- 1 bunch of green beans, ends cut off

- Add a little cayenne pepper and stir.
- Cook vegetables for about 16 minutes, stirring at 8-minute intervals.
- As soon as the vegetables are lightly browned, remove from heat and serve.

24) Crockpot Summer Vegetables

Preparation time: **Cooking time:** **Servings: 6**

Ingredients:
- 1 tablespoon chopped thyme, fresh
- 2 tablespoons chopped basil, fresh
- ½ cup olive oil
- Juice of 1 lemon
- 1 cup sliced mushrooms

Ingredients:
- 2 ½ cups sliced zucchini
- 2 cups sliced bell bell pepper, yellow
- 1 ½ cup chopped onions
- 1 cup chopped cherry tomatoes
- 2 cups of sliced okra

Directions:
- Mix the vegetables in a bowl, then stir in the olive oil and lemon juice in a separate bowl.
- Stir in the thyme and basil and place the vegetables in a slow stove.
- Cover with marinade and stir to coat.
- Cook vegetables over high heat for 3 hours, stirring every hour.
- Once cooked, serve and enjoy.

25) Brazilian Cabbage

Preparation time: **Cooking time:** **Servings: 2**

Ingredients:
- Juice of 1/2 lime
- 1/4 teaspoon cayenne pepper
- 1/4 teaspoon salt

Ingredients:
- 2 bunches of cabbage, thin strips
- 2 fennel bulbs, peeled, cut and crushed
- 2 tablespoons of olive oil

Directions:
- Remove crusts from cabbage, stack leaf halves and slice cabbage.
- Crush the fennel bulbs using the flat end of a chef's knife or a pestle and mortar.
- In a large skillet, heat the olive oil on medium for a minute and then add the fennel.
- Sauté for 1 minute or until aromatic, and then add the cayenne pepper, salt and cabbage.
- Lower the heat to medium low and sauté to soften the greens and get a vibrant color or about 3-4 minutes.
- Then squeeze in the lime juice and add more salt and cayenne pepper if needed. Serve and enjoy.

26) Algae Wraps With Quinoa And Vegetables

Preparation time: **Cooking time:** **Servings: 2 rolls**

Ingredients:
- 1 tablespoon sesame seed oil
- 1 tablespoon raw sesame seeds
- 1 teaspoon fresh ginger root, finely grated
- 1 teaspoon fresh red chili pepper with seeds and finely chopped
- 1 finely chopped fennel bulb

Ingredients:
- ¼ cup finely chopped fresh culantro leaves
- ¼ cup of raw cucumber sticks
- ¼ cup raw parsnips
- ½ cup of cooked quinoa

Directions:
- Spread 2 sheets of nori individually on a work surface.
- Mix quinoa with chili, ginger, fennel, seeds and culantro leaves.
- In this mixture, add the sesame seed oil and mix well.
- Spread the seed and quinoa mixture between two sheets of nori, placing it along the edge of each sheet.
- Top the quinoa mixture with the parsnip sticks and cucumber. Now roll up the sheets and gently wrap the contents.
- If you want, you can slide the nori rolls around until they look like sushi rolls.

27) Lettuce Wraps

Preparation time: **Cooking time:** **Servings: 4 wrappers**

Ingredients:
- ½ cup coarsely chopped raw walnuts
- ½ cup fresh strawberries, sliced
- ½ of a ripe avocado, pitted and cut into slices

Directions:
- Spread the lettuce leaves out on a work surface or kitchen plate.
- Divide the green beans among the individual lettuce leaves, placing them at a 90-degree angle to the edge.
- Now divide the avocado slices between the individual lettuce leaves placing them on top of the spears.

Ingredients:
- 1 cup raw green beans
- 4 large lettuce leaves

- Also divide the berries among the individual lettuce leaves and place them on top of the avocado.
- Then divide the nuts between the lettuce leaves and place them on top of the berries.
- Finally, roll up the leaves and wrap the entire contents.

28) Rainbow Salad With Meyer Lemon Dressing

Preparation time: **Cooking time:** **Servings: 4**

Ingredients:
- 1/2 avocado, sliced
- Micro green or sprouts
- 1 cup of pea shoots
- ½ yellow bell pepper, sliced
- 1/8 red onion, thinly sliced
- ½ cup diced cherry tomatoes
- 1 parsnip, ribbon with peeler
- Arugula and other vegetables
- Chopped or chipped raw nuts

Directions:
- Place a handful of arugula in each bowl.
- Add the rest of the vegetables and then the micro greens and pea shoots.
- Then, top with the walnuts and set aside.

Ingredients:
For the dressing
- 1 tablespoon of agave sugar
- 1/16 teaspoon of sea salt
- 1/6 cup of cold-pressed extra virgin olive oil
- 3 stalks of fresh dill
- 3 basil leaves
- 3/4 teaspoon of chopped red onion
- ½ avocado
- 1 Meyer lemon, squeezed

- Now move the ingredients for the dressing to a blender and blend until smooth and creamy.
- Pour the dressing into a serving bowl and then pour it over the salad and enjoy!

29) Alkaline Quinoa & Hummus Wraps

Preparation time: **Cooking time:** **Servings: 4 wrappers**

Ingredients:
- 1 cup avocado
- 1 cup hummus
- 1 cup of quinoa
- 1/2 cup parsnips

Directions:
- Place 1 cup of quinoa in a skillet with 2 cups of water. Bring the water to a boil and lower the heat to a simmer until the quinoa is soft and the water has evaporated.
- Cut the cabbage leaves from the plant, wash them and arrange them like a regular wrap. Spread hummus on each cabbage to help hold the other ingredients in place.

Ingredients:
- 1/2 cup of lettuce
- 1/2 cup of sprouts
- 4 large baby cabbage

- Now slice and place the avocado in a line from top to bottom and down the center of the cabbage leaf.
- Once done, place the quinoa evenly between the cabbage leaves and fill with the rest of the ingredients.
- Finally wrap the leaf. Fold it down and then roll it up. Consider using a toothpick to help keep things in place.

30) Grilled Zucchini Salad

Preparation time: **Cooking time:**   **Servings: 2**

Ingredients:
- 3 ounces of watercress
- 6 zucchinis
- Sea Salt
- Chili pepper and mint dressing:
- 6 tablespoons of extra virgin olive oil

Directions:
- Clean the watercress and zucchini. Then slice the zucchini into thin strips. Salt the strips and let them soften slightly in the salt.
- Meanwhile, start preparing the dressing. Wash the basil leaves, chili pepper and lemon and set aside.
- Discard the seeds of the chili and chop well. Then shred the leaves and set aside.
- In a bowl, whisk together the olive oil, basil, red pepper and lemon zest and then season with cayenne pepper and salt.

Ingredients:
- ½ cup of fresh basil leaves
- 1 red hot pepper
- Zest and juice of 1/2 lemon
- Cayenne Pepper
- Halls
- Now place the watercress in a serving dish.
- Fire up your barbecue for direct heat at 220 degrees F. Place the salt-softened strips on a rack and close the lid.
- Now grill the zucchini until spots develop, or for about 3 to 4 minutes per side.
- Then remove them from the grill and let them cool. To serve, place the zucchini on the watercress and then pour the dressing over it.

31) Creamy Cabbage Salad With Avocado And Tomato

Preparation time: **Cooking time:**   **Servings: 2**

Ingredients:
- 1/2 teaspoon of cayenne pepper
- 1 tablespoon of agave syrup
- 1 funnel-shaped bulb, chopped
- Juice of 1 lime

Directions:
- Clean and chop the tomatoes and cabbage and then place them in a bowl or large glass bowl.
- Then peel the avocado and place it in the bowl.

Ingredients:
- ½ cup chopped cherry tomatoes
- 1 medium ripe avocado
- 2 large handfuls of cabbage

- Squeeze the lime and now add it along with the rest of the ingredients into the mixing bowl.
- Rub the ingredients together and serve the salad.

32) Rice With Sesame And Ginger

Preparation time: **Cooking time:**   **Servings: 4**

Ingredients:
- 1/2 teaspoon celtic sea salt
- 2 teaspoons of fresh lime juice
- ½ cup culantro, finely chopped
- 4 cups mushrooms (any kind except shiitake), finely chopped
- 6 green onions, finely chopped
- 1 fennel bulb, chopped

Directions:
- Heat oil in a deep skillet or wok over medium-high heat.
- Once hot, sauté the mushrooms, green onions, fennel, ginger and chili along with a little salt until soft and combined, or for about 5 minutes.

Ingredients:
- 2 tablespoons fresh chopped ginger
- 1 small green chili pepper, ribbed, seeded and chopped
- 2 tablespoons of toasted sesame oil
- 2 tablespoons of grape oil
- 1 cup of cooked wild rice

- Add the tamari and rice and keep on the heat for another 2-3 minutes.
- Add the lime juice, culantro and ¼ teaspoon salt and taste.

33) Macaroni And 'Cheese

Preparation time: 20 minutes. **Cooking time**: 50 minutes. **Servings**: 8-10

Ingredients:
- 12 ounces of any alkaline pasta
- 1/4 cup of chickpea flour
- 1 cup of raw Brazil Nuts
- 1/2 teaspoon of Achiote Ground
- 2 teaspoons of onion powder

Directions:
- Put the Brazil Nuts in a lunch bowl and add the soy water. Place on the right side.
- Coook your favorite alkaline pasta.
- Preheat our oven to 350 degrees Fahrenheit.
- Place the processed dough in an oven dish and pour a little semi-fat oil to prevent it from sticking to the bread.

Ingredients:
- 1 teaspoon of Pure Sea Salt
- 2 teaspoons of Oil Sed Grape
- 1 cup of milk Homemade Hempsed
- 1 cup of spring water + an addition of juice of 1/2 Key Lime
- Add all ingredients to a blender and blend 2 to 4 minutes until ready.
- Pour the Brazil nut sauce over the macaroni and mix well.
- Place the pan in the oven and bake for about 30 minutes.
- Serve and enjoy your Macaroni and 'Cheese'!
- Useful Tips:
- If you don't have Homemad Hempsed Milk milk, add Coconut Milk insted. If you want to make the dish crispy, cook it for about 5 minutes.

34) Creamy Kamut Pasta

Preparation time: 25 minutes. **Cooking time**: 50 Minutes. **Servings**: 6

Ingredients:

Pasta:
- 12 ounces of Kamut Spaghetti
- 1 tablespoon of tarragon
- 1 teaspoon of Onion Powder.
- 1 teaspoon of pure marine Salt
- 2 tablespoons of Grape Seed Oil 6 to 8 cups of Spring Water (for boiling the pasta)

Sauce:
- 2 cups of chopped Kale
- 12 Cherry chopped tomatoes
- 1/2 diced Onion
- 2 sliced mushrooms

Directions:
- Pasta:
- In a large saucepan, bring the Spring Water to a boil. Add the Pure Sea Salt to taste.
- Add Kamut noodles to boiling water. Cook for about 8-10 minutes until noodles are dry.
- Drink the pasta and put it in a glass. Add the pure sea salt, peanut butter, onion powder and ground olive oil to maximize the float.
- Mix the mixture well.
- Sauce:
- Add 1 tablespoon of Grape Seed Oil to a medium saucepan and heat over medium heat.
- Add sliced Mushrooms and diced Onions to top. Cook 3 to 5 minutes, stirring.
- Sprinkle 1/4 teaspoon of pure sea salt and 1/8 teaspoon of Cayenne over the vegetables and stir.

Ingredients:
- 1/4 cup of Garbanzo Bean Flour
- 2 teaspoons of Onion Powder
- 1 tablespoon of Oregano
- 1 teaspoon of Tarragon
- 1 teaspoon of Basil
- 1/4 teaspoon of Pure Sea Salt + extra 1/2 teaspoon
- 1/8 teaspoon of Cayenne Powder + extra 1/8 teaspoon
- 2 tablespoons of Grape Seed Oil
- 2 cups of coconut Milk
- 2 cups of Spring Water

- Place the chickpea flour and another tablespoon of cereal oil in the bowl. Stir until everything is well combined and there is no trace of dry flour.
- Add the nut milk, soybean oil, 1/2 teaspoon of Pure Sea Salt, Onion Powder, Oregano, Tarragon, and Basil and stir.
- Simmer for 20 minutes until slightly thickened.
- Add the cooked pasta, chopped tomatoes and cabbage to the pot. Soak 3 to 5 minutes until cabbage has dried and remove from heat.
- Serve and enjoy your Creamy Kamut Pasta!
- Helpful Hints:
- Don't go swimming on your own time!
- Creamy Kamut Pasta will keep in the refrigerator for 3-4 days.

35) Basil Avocado Pasta

Preparation time: 10 minutes.　　**Cooking time:** 20 Minutes.　　**Servings:** 4

Ingredients:
- 4 cups of cooked Spelt pasta
- 1 medium diced Avocado
- 2 cups of halved Cherry Tomatoes
- 1 fresh basil chopped

Directions:
- Place the cooked meat in a large container.
- Add the Avocado dicedo, Cherry Tomatoes and chopped Basil to the bowl.
- Hold all ingredients in place until removed.

Ingredients:
- 1 teaspoon of Agave Syrup
- 1 tablespoon of Key Lime Juice.
- 1/4 cup o of olive oil

- Mix the agave syrup, olive oil and Pure Sea Salt a Key Lime in a separate bowl.
- Pour into container and stir until well bottled.
- Enjoy your avocado pasta Basil!

36) Jamaican Jerk Patties

Preparation time: 35 minutes.　　**Cooking time:** 1 hour.　　**Servings:** 3-4

Ingredients:
- Filling:
- 1 cup of cooked Garbanzo Beans
- 1/2 bell pepper cup, diced
- 1 prune
- 2 cups of chopped Mushroms
- 1 cup of chopped Butternut Squash
- 1/2 cup of diced Onions
- 1 tablespoon of onion Powder
- 1 teaspoon of Ginger
- 2 teaspoons of thyme
- 1 tablespoon of Agave Syrup
- 1/2 teaspoon of Cayenne Powder
- 1 teaspoon of Allspice.

Directions:
- Preheat the oven to 350 degrees Fahrenheit.
- Add all the vegetables, excluding the Cherry Tomatoes, to a refrigerator. Wipe a few times to make them stiffer.
- Mix vegetables with seasonings and tomatoes in a cup. This constitutes the filling for the patties.
- In a separate glass jar, place the Spelt Flour, Grape Seed Oil and seasonings.
- Pour in 1/2 quart of water and knead the dough into a loaf, adding more water or flour if necessary.
- Allow to rest for 5 to 10 minutes. Knead for a few minutes and then divide into 8 parts.

Ingredients:
- 1/4 teaspoon of cloves
- 1 teaspoon of Pure Sea Salt
- Crust:
- 1 1/2 cups of Spelt Flour
- 1/4 cup of Aquafaba
- 1 teaspoon of Pure Sea Salt
- 1/8 teaspoon of Ginger powder
- 1 teaspoon of Onion Powder.
- 1 tablespoon of Grape Seed Oil
- 1 cup of spring water

- Make a piece of wood into a stack and then roll the stack into a 6-7 cm box.
- Take a circular dough and put 1/2 cup of filling in the center. Brush all the edges of the dough with the Aquafaba, cover it and slide the edge with a knife.
- Repeat step 8 until all dough cirles are filled.
- Lightly coat a baking sheet with a little Grape Seed Oil.
- Bake the stuffed meatballs for about 25-30 minutes until golden brown.
- Serve and enjoy your Jamican Jerk Patties!
- Tips useful:
- You can serve Jamaican Jerk Patties with our Fragrant Tomato Sauce.

37) Kamut Patties

Preparation time: 15 minutes. **Cooking time:** 30 minutes. **Servings:** 3-4

Ingredients:
- 3 cups of cooked Kamut Cereal
- 1 cup of chopped Red Onions
- 1 cup of green peppers and Yellow chopped
- 1 cup of Spelt Flour
- ½ cup of Homemade Hempseed Milk
- 1 tablespoon of Basil

Directions:
- Combine the vegetables, hemp seed milk, hemp seed flour and kamut milk in a large bowl.
- Put 1/2 cup of spelt flour in the bowl and mix well. Keep adding more flour until you can form a patties shape.
- Heat soybean oil in a skillet over medium heat. Form patties from the mixture and place in the oven.

Ingredients:
- ½ teaspoon of Cayenne Powder
- 1 tablespoon of Oregano
- 1 tablespoon of Onion Powder.
- 1 teaspoon of salt Pure Sea
- 2 tablespoons of Grade Seed Oil

- Coook patties for about 4 or 5 minutes on each side.
- Serve and enjoy your kamut meatballs!
- Tips useful:
- If you don't have Spelt flour, add Gärbazo Bean Flour instead flour.
- You can enjoy kamut meatballs with our French "Cheese" or French tomato sauce.

38) Mushroom Burgers Portobello

Preparation time: 25 minutes. **Cooking time:** 50 Minutes. **Servings:** 2

Ingredients:
- 2 cups Portobello Mushrom caps
- 1 sliced Avocado
- 1 sliced Plum Tomatoes
- 1 cup of torn Lettuce
- 1 cup of Purslane

Directions:
- Set your oven to 425 degrees Fahrenheit.
- Remove the mushroom and cut 1/2 inch off the top slice, as if you were slicing a sandwich.
- In a medium bowl mix the alder powder, cinnamon, oregano, olive oil and butter.
- Cover a sheet of baking paper and brush with the grape oil to prevent sticking.
- Place mushroom caps on a baking sheet and brush with the prepared marinade. Marinate for 10 minutes before starting to bake.
- Bake for 10 minutes until brown, then unmold. Continue baking for another 10 minutes.

Ingredients:
- 1/2 teaspoon of Cayenne
- 1 teaspoon of Oregano.
- 2 teaspoons of Basil
- 3 tablespoons of olive oil

- Lay out the mushrom cap on a serving dish. This will serve as the basis for the mushroom burger.
- On it are avocado, tomatoes, lettuce and puree.
- Cover the burger with another mushrom capm. Repeat steps 7 and 8 with the mushrooms and vermicelli.
- Feel and enjoy our Portobello Mushroom Burgers!
- Useful Tips:
- You can add any type of lettuce, exotic lettuce, chives and other ingredients to suit your taste.
- You can serve Portobello Mushroom Burgers with our "Chese" Sauce or Fragrant Tomato Sauce.

39) Healthy Fried-Rice

Preparation time: 15 minutes. **Cooking time:** 50 minutes. **Servings:** 2

Ingredients:
- 1 cup of cooked Wild Rice
- 1/2 cup of sliced Mushrooms
- 1/2 cup of cubed Zucchini
- 1/2 cup of cubed Bell Peppers

Directions:
- Heat the soybean oil in a medium skillet over medium heat.
- Add the onion diced to the skillet and sauté until golden brown.
- Add the mushrooms, Zucchini and Peppers bell and coook for 5 more minutes. The vegetables should get a little softer.

234kcal. Fat: 7g. Carbs: 13g. Protein: 11g.

Ingredients:
- 1/4 onion, diced
- Pure Sea Salt, a taste
- Cayenne Powder, per taste
- 1/2 tablespoon of Grape Seed Oil

- Add the Wild Rice boiled to the oven and continue working until lightly browned.
- Serve and enjoy your Healthy Fried-Rice!
- Useful Tips:
- If you want, you can use cooked quinoa instead.

40) *Veg-Meatballs*

Preparation time: 10 minutes.   **Cooking time**: 30 minutes   **Servings**: 7-9

Ingredients:
- 1 1/2 cups of Garbanzo Beans cooked
- 1 cup of Garbanzo Bean Flour
- 2 cups of Mushrooms
- 1/4 cup of diced Green Peppers
- 1/2 cup of diced Onions
- 2 teaspoons of Oregano
- 1 tablespoon of Onion Powder
- 2 teaspoons of Basil
- 1 teaspoon of Fennel Powder

Ingredients:
- 1 teaspoon of Dill
- 1 teaspoon of Savory
- 1 teaspoon of Sage
- 1/2 teaspoon of Ginger Powder 1/2 teaspoon of Ground Cloves
- 1 teaspoon of Pure Sea Salt
- 1/2 teaspoon of cayenne powder
- 6 cups by Fragrant Tomato Sauce
- 2 tablespoons or semi-fat oil

Directions:
- Place the cooked mushrooms, Garbanzo beans, onions, green peppers and seasonings into a processor. Blend well for 1 minute.
- Add dough to a large bowl and mix with Garrbazo Bean Flour. Cut into a ball of dough. If they do not form, add more sugar.
- Turn off the oven and let it rest for a couple of minutes.
- Add Grape Seed Oil to a saucepan and heat over low heat.
- Place a couple of patties on the baking sheet. Bake for 2 minutes on each side.
- Add Fragrant Tomato Sauce to the meatballs and simmer for 5 minutes.
- Serve and enjoy your Meatballs!
- Useful Tips:
- You can use it with our flatbread or Homemade bread dough.

Chapter 4 -   Dinner Recipes

41) Cabbage, Soursop And Zucchini Soup

Preparation time: 5 minutes **Cooking time:** 45 minutes **Servings:** 2

Ingredients:
- 1 cup chopped cabbage
- 2 soursop leaves, rinsed, torn in half
- ½ cup summer squash cubes
- 1 cup of chayote pumpkin cubes
- ½ cup of zucchini cubes
- ½ cup wild rice
- ½ cup diced white onions

Directions:
- Take a medium saucepan, place it over medium-high heat, add the soursop leaves, pour in 1 1/2 cups of water and boil for 15 minutes, covering the saucepan with a lid.

Ingredients:
- 1 cup diced green peppers
- 2 teaspoons of sea salt
- ½ tablespoon of basil
- ¼ teaspoon cayenne pepper
- ½ tablespoon of oregano
- 6 cups of spring water

- Once done, remove the gutters from the broth, turn the heat up to medium, add the remaining ingredients to the pot, stir until combined, and then cook for 30 minutes or more until cooked through.
- Serve immediately.

42) Green Chickpea Soup

Preparation time: 5 minutes **Cooking time:** 25 minutes **Servings:** 2

Ingredients:
- ½ cup of cooked chickpeas
- ½ of a medium white onion, peeled, diced
- ½ of a large zucchini, chopped
- 1 cup of kale leaves
- 1 cup of pumpkin cubes

Directions:
- Take a saucepan, place it over medium-high heat, pour in the ¼ cup of broth, add the zucchini, onion and thyme and cook for 4 minutes.

Ingredients:
- ¾ teaspoon salt
- ¾ tablespoon chopped thyme, fresh
- ¾ tablespoon tarragon, fresh
- 2 cups of vegetable broth, homemade
- 1½ cups of spring water

- Pour in the remaining broth and water, bring to a boil, lower the heat, and then simmer for 10-15 minutes until tender.
- Add the remaining ingredients, stir until combined, and then continue cooking for 10 minutes or more, until cooked through.
- Serve immediately.

43) Green Zucchini Soup

Preparation time: 10 minutes **Cooking time:** 10 minutes **Servings:** 2

Ingredients:
- 2 cups of leafy greens
- 1 small zucchini, sliced
- 1 small white onion, peeled, sliced
- 1 medium green bell pepper, with core, cut into slices

Directions:
- Take a medium saucepan, put it on medium heat, add all the ingredients, stir until combined, and then cook for 5-10 minutes until the vegetables become tender-crispy.

Ingredients:
- 2 ½ cups of spring water
- ¾ teaspoon salt
- ¼ teaspoon cayenne pepper
- 1 teaspoon of dried basil

- Remove the pot from the heat, blend the soup with an immersion blender and then serve.

44) Kamut Vegetable Soup With Tarragon

Preparation time: 5 minutes **Cooking time:** 32 minutes **Servings:** 2

Ingredients:
- ✓ 6 tablespoons of kamut berries
- ✓ 1 cup chopped white onion
- ✓ ½ cup chopped pumpkin
- ✓ ½ cup of cooked chickpeas
- ✓ 1 cup of homemade vegetable broth
- ✓ ¼ teaspoon cayenne pepper

Directions:
- ❖ Place the kamut in a small bowl, pour in the boiling water and let it sit for 30 minutes.
- ❖ Then take a medium saucepan, put it over medium heat, add the oil and when hot, add the onion, stir in the thyme and tarragon and then cook for 5 minutes until tender.

Ingredients:
- ✓ ½ tablespoon of chopped tarragon
- ✓ 1 bay leaf
- ✓ 1 teaspoon of chopped thyme
- ✓ 1 tablespoon of olive oil
- ✓ 1 cup of spring water, boiling

- ❖ Drain the kamut, add it to the pot, add the bay leaf, pour in the vegetable stock and bring to a boil.
- ❖ Cover the pot with its lid, simmer for 20-30 minutes, then stir in the cayenne pepper and cook for 5 minutes.
- ❖ Remove the bay leaf, add the chickpeas and cook for 2 minutes.
- ❖ Serve immediately.

45) Pumpkin Soup With Basil

Preparation time: 5 minutes **Cooking time:** 25 minutes **Servings:** 2

Ingredients:
- ✓ ½ of a medium white onion, peeled, cut into cubes
- ✓ 2 cups cubed pumpkin
- ✓ ¼ cup of basil leaves
- ✓ ½ cup coconut cream softener jelly

Directions:
- ❖ Take a medium saucepan, put it over medium heat, add the oil and when hot, add the onion, and then cook for 5 minutes or until softened.
- ❖ Add the squash, cook for 10 minutes until golden brown and beginning to soften, pour in the vegetable broth, season with salt and pepper and then bring the soup to a boil.

Ingredients:
- ✓ ⅛ teaspoon sea salt
- ✓ ⅛ teaspoon of cayenne pepper
- ✓ 1 tablespoon of grape oil
- ✓ 1 cup of homemade vegetable broth

- ❖ Turn the heat to medium and simmer the soup for 10 minutes until the squash becomes very soft.
- ❖ Remove the pan from the heat, blend with an immersion blender until smooth, and then garnish with the basil.
- ❖ Serve immediately.

46) Coconut Mushroom Soup

Preparation time: 5 minutes **Cooking time:** 20 minutes **Servings:** 2

Ingredients:
- ✓ 2 cups of baby Bella mushrooms, diced
- ✓ ½ cup diced red onions
- ✓ 1 cup of vegetable broth
- ✓ 1½ cups of soft coconut milk jelly

Directions:
- ❖ Take a medium saucepan, put it over medium-high heat, add the oil and when hot, add the onion, mushrooms, season with salt and pepper, and then cook for 3 to 4 minutes until the vegetables become tender.

Ingredients:
- ✓ ½ teaspoon of sea salt
- ✓ ¼ teaspoon cayenne pepper
- ✓ 2 teaspoons of grape oil

- ❖ Then add the soy sauce, pour in the milk and broth, stir until combined and bring to a boil.
- ❖ Turn the heat to medium-low and simmer the soup for 15 minutes until it has thickened to the desired level.
- ❖ Serve immediately.

47) Onion And Pumpkin Soup

Preparation time: 5 minutes **Cooking time**: 35 minutes **Servings: 2**

Ingredients:
- 2 large white onions, peeled, sliced
- ½ cup diced pumpkin
- 1 sprig of thyme
- 1 tablespoon of grape oil

Directions:
- Take a medium saucepan, put it over medium heat, add the oil and when hot, add the onion and cook for 10 minutes.
- Add the sprig of thyme, lower the heat and cook the onions for 15-20 minutes until soft, covering the pan with its lid.

Ingredients:
- 2 cups of spring water
- ½ teaspoon salt
- ¼ teaspoon cayenne pepper

- Add remaining ingredients, stir until combined and simmer for 5 minutes.
- Pour the soup into bowls and then serve.

48) Chayote Mushroom And Hemp Milk Stew

Preparation time: 10 minutes **Cooking time**: 40 minutes **Servings: 2**

Ingredients:
- ⅔ cup of chayote pumpkin cubes
- 1 cup sliced mushrooms
- ⅓ cup of diced white onions
- ½ cup of chickpea flour
- ⅓ cup of vegetable broth, homemade
- ⅓ tablespoon of onion powder
- ⅔ teaspoon of sea salt

Directions:
- Take a medium saucepan, put it over medium-high heat, add the oil and when it's hot, add the onion and mushrooms, and then cook for 5 minutes.
- Bring the heat to medium, pour in 1 cup of the water, milk and broth, add the chayote and all the seasonings, stir until combined, and then bring everything to a boil, covering the pot with the lid.

Ingredients:
- ⅔ teaspoon dried basil
- ⅓ teaspoon crushed red pepper
- 2 cups of spring water
- ½ tablespoon of grape oil
- ⅓ cup of hemp milk, homemade

- Pour remaining water into a food processor, add chickpea flour, pulse until combined, add to pot and then blend until combined.
- Lower the heat, simmer for 30 minutes, and then serve.

49) Coconut Soup With Butternut Squash

Preparation time: 5 minutes **Cooking time**: 15 minutes **Servings: 2**

Ingredients:
- 2 medium-sized pumpkins, peeled, seeds removed and cut into pieces
- 1 medium white onion, peeled, chopped
- 2 cups of soft coconut milk jelly

Directions:
- Take a large saucepan, place it over medium-high heat, pour in the water and bring it to a boil.
- Stir in salt and add the vegetables and then cook for 5-10 minutes until the vegetables become tender.

Ingredients:
- ⅔ teaspoon of sea salt
- 1 cup of spring water

- Remove the pan from the heat, add the milk and then blend with an immersion blender until smooth.
- Serve immediately

50) Mushroom And Tomato Coconut Soup

Preparation time: 5 minutes　　**Cooking time:** 10 minutes　　**Servings:** 2

Ingredients:
- 1½ cups sliced mushrooms
- 8 cherry tomatoes, chopped
- 1 medium onion, peeled, sliced
- ¾ cup of vegetable broth, homemade
- 6 teaspoons of spice mixture

Ingredients:
- ¼ teaspoon salt
- ½ tablespoon of grape oil
- ¼ teaspoon cayenne pepper
- ¾ cup tomato sauce, alkaline
- 6 tablespoons of soft coconut milk jelly

Directions:
- Take a large skillet, put it over medium heat, add the oil and heat, add the onion, and then cook for 5 minutes until golden brown.
- Add the spice mix, add the remaining ingredients to the pan except the okra, stir until combined, and then bring the mixture to a simmer.
- Add mushrooms, stir until combined and cook for 10-15 minutes over medium-low heat until cooked through.
- Serve immediately

51) Curried Cabbage And Chickpeas

Preparation time: 5 minutes　　**Cooking time:** 10 minutes　　**Servings:** 2

Ingredients:
- 2 cups of cooked chickpeas
- ⅔ teaspoon of salt
- 1 cup of kale leaves

Ingredients:
- ⅔ cup of coconut cream in soft jelly
- 2 tablespoons of grape oil
- ⅓ teaspoon cayenne pepper

Directions:
- Turn on the oven, then set it to 425°F (220°C) and let it preheat.
- Then take a medium baking dish, spread out the chickpeas, drizzle with 1 tablespoon of oil, sprinkle with all the seasonings and then bake for 15 minutes until roasted.
- Then take a skillet, put it over medium heat, add the remaining oil and when hot, add the cabbage and cook for 5 minutes.
- Add the roasted chickpeas, pour in the cream, stir until combined and then simmer for 4 minutes, mashing the chickpeas slightly.
- Serve immediately.

52) Coconut And Cashew Soup With Tarragon

Preparation time: 10 minutes　　**Cooking time:** 10 minutes　　**Servings:** 1 to 2

Ingredients:
- 1 tablespoon avocado oil
- ½ cup diced onion
- 3 garlic cloves, crushed
- ¼ plus ⅛ teaspoon sea salt
- ¼ plus ⅛ teaspoon freshly ground black pepper

Ingredients:
- 1 (13.5-ounce / 383-g) can of whole coconut milk
- 1 tablespoon freshly squeezed lemon juice
- ½ cup raw cashews
- 1 celery stalk
- 2 tablespoons fresh tarragon chopped

Directions:
- In a medium skillet over medium-high heat, heat the avocado oil. Add the onion, garlic, salt and pepper and sauté for 3-5 minutes, or until the onion is soft.
- In a high-speed blender, blend together the coconut milk, lemon juice, cashews, celery and tarragon with the onion mixture until smooth. Adjust seasonings as needed.
- Pour into 1 large or 2 small bowls and enjoy immediately, or transfer to a medium saucepan and heat over low heat for 3-5 minutes before serving.

53) Cucumber And Zucchini Soup

Preparation time: 5 minutes **Cooking time:** 0 minutes **Servings:** 1 to 2

Ingredients:
- 1 cucumber, peeled
- ½ zucchini, peeled
- 1 tablespoon freshly squeezed lime juice

Directions:
- In a blender, blend together the cucumber, zucchini, lime juice, cilantro, garlic and salt until well combined. Add more salt, if needed.

Ingredients:
- 1 tablespoon of fresh coriander leaves
- 1 garlic clove, crushed
- ¼ teaspoon of sea salt
- Pour into 1 large or 2 small bowls and enjoy immediately, or refrigerate for 15-20 minutes to chill before serving.

54) Coconut Soup With Jalapeno And Lime

Preparation time: 5 minutes **Cooking time:** 5 minutes **Servings:** 2

Ingredients:
- 2 tablespoons of avocado oil
- ½ cup diced onions
- 3 garlic cloves, crushed
- ¼ teaspoon of sea salt

Directions:
- In a medium skillet over medium-high heat, heat the avocado oil. Add the onion, garlic and salt, and sauté for 3-5 minutes, or until the onions are soft.

Ingredients:
- 1 (13.5-ounce / 383-g) can of whole coconut milk
- 1 tablespoon freshly squeezed lime juice
- ½ to 1 jalapeño
- 2 tablespoons of fresh coriander leaves
- In a blender, blend together the coconut milk, lime juice, jalapeño and cilantro with the onion mixture until creamy.
- Pour into 1 large or 2 small bowls and enjoy.

55) Watermelon And Jalapeno Gazpacho

Preparation time: 5 minutes **Cooking time:** 0 minutes **Servings:** 1 to 2

Ingredients:
- 2 cups of diced watermelon
- ¼ cup diced onion
- ¼ cup of packed coriander leaves

Directions:
- In a blender or food processor, give a pulse to combine the watermelon, onion, cilantro, jalapeño and lime juice just enough to break up the ingredients, leaving them chopped very finely and being careful not to over process them.

57 | Fat: 0.3g | Protein: 1.2g | Carbohydrates: 14.4g | Fiber: 1.1g

Ingredients:
- ½ to 1 jalapeño
- 2 tablespoons freshly squeezed lime juice

- Pour into 1 large or 2 small bowls and enjoy.
- Per serving

56) Carrot And Fennel Soup

Preparation time: 10 minutes **Cooking time:** 30 minutes **Servings:** 2 to 1

Ingredients:
- 6 carrots
- 1 cup chopped onion
- 1 fennel bulb, diced
- 2 garlic cloves, crushed

Directions:
- Preheat the oven to 400°F (205°C). Line a baking sheet with baking paper.
- Cut carrots into thirds and then cut each third in half. Transfer to a medium bowl.
- Add the onion, fennel, garlic and avocado oil and toss to coat. Season with the salt and pepper and toss again.

Ingredients:
- 2 tablespoons of avocado oil
- 1 teaspoon of sea salt
- 1 teaspoon of freshly ground black pepper
- 2 cups almond milk, more if desired
- Transfer the vegetables to the prepared baking sheet and roast for 30 minutes.
- Remove from oven and allow vegetables to cool.
- In a high-speed blender, blend together the almond milk and roasted vegetables until creamy and smooth. Adjust seasonings, if necessary, and add more milk if you prefer a thinner consistency.
- Pour into 2 large or 4 small bowls and enjoy.

57) Coconut Stew With Lentils And Herb Potatoes

Preparation time: 10 minutes **Cooking time**: 30 minutes **Servings**: 4

Ingredients:
- 2 tablespoons of avocado oil
- ½ cup diced onion
- 2 garlic cloves, crushed
- 1 to 1½ teaspoons of sea salt
- 1 teaspoon of freshly ground black pepper
- 1 cup of dried lentils
- 2 carrots, sliced

Directions:
- In a large soup pot over medium-high heat, heat the avocado oil. Add the onion, garlic, salt and pepper, and sauté for 3-5 minutes, or until the onion is soft.
- Add the lentils, carrots, potato, celery, oregano, tarragon and 2½ cups of vegetable stock and stir.

Ingredients:
- 1 cup potatoes, peeled and diced
- 1 celery stalk, diced
- 2 sprigs of fresh oregano, chopped
- 2 sprigs fresh tarragon, chopped
- 5 cups vegetable stock, divided
- 1 (13.5-ounce / 383-g) can of whole coconut milk

- Bring to a boil, reduce the heat to medium-low and cook, stirring often and adding more vegetable stock a half cup at a time to make sure there is enough liquid to cook the lentils and potatoes, for 20-25 minutes, or until the potatoes and lentils are soft.
- Remove from heat and stir in coconut milk. Pour into 4 soup bowls and enjoy.

58) Cauliflower And Roasted Garlic Soup

Preparation time: 10 minutes **Cooking time**: 35 minutes **Servings**: 1 to 2

Ingredients:
- 4 cups chopped cauliflower florets
- 5 garlic cloves
- 1½ tablespoons of avocado oil
- ¾ teaspoon of sea salt

Directions:
- Preheat the oven to 450°F (235°C). Line a baking sheet with baking paper.
- In a medium bowl, toss the cauliflower and garlic with the avocado oil. Season with the salt and pepper and toss again.
- Transfer to prepared baking sheet and roast for 30 minutes. Cool before adding to blender.

Ingredients:
- ½ teaspoon of freshly ground black pepper
- 1 cup of almond milk
- 1 cup vegetable stock, more if desired

- In a high-speed blender, whisk together the cooled vegetables, almond milk, and vegetable broth until smooth. Adjust the salt and pepper, if necessary, and add more vegetable broth if you prefer a thinner consistency.
- Transfer to a medium saucepan and heat slightly over medium-low heat for 3-5 minutes.
- Pour into 1 large or 2 small bowls and enjoy.

59) Carrot And Potato Stew With Herbs

Preparation time: 10 minutes **Cooking time**: 50 minutes **Servings**: 4 people

Ingredients:
- 1 tablespoon avocado oil
- 1 cup onion, diced
- 2 garlic cloves, crushed
- 1 teaspoon of sea salt
- 1 teaspoon of freshly ground black pepper
- 3 cups vegetable stock, more if desired

Directions:
- In a medium saucepan over medium heat, heat the avocado oil. Add the onion, garlic, salt and pepper, and sauté for 2 to 3 minutes, or until the onion is soft.
- Add the vegetable stock, water, carrot, potato, celery, oregano and bay leaf and stir. Bring to a boil, reduce heat to medium-low and cook for 30-45 minutes, or until potatoes and carrots are soft.

Ingredients:
- 2 cups of water, plus more if desired
- 3 cups of sliced carrots
- 1 large potato, cubed
- 2 stalks of celery, diced
- 1 teaspoon of dried oregano
- 1 dried bay leaf

- Adjust seasonings, if necessary, and add more water or vegetable broth if you prefer a softer consistency, in half-cup increments.
- Pour into 4 soup bowls and enjoy.

60) Berry And Mint Soup

Preparation time: 5 minutes **Cooking time**: 0 minutes **Servings: 1 to 2**

Ingredients:
- ¼ cup unrefined whole cane sugar, such as Sucanat
- ¼ cup water, more if desired
- 1 cup mixed berries (raspberries, blackberries, blueberries)

Ingredients:
- ½ cup of water
- 1 teaspoon of freshly squeezed lemon juice
- 8 fresh mint leaves

Directions:
- In a small saucepan over medium-low heat, heat sugar and water, stirring constantly for 1 to 2 minutes, until sugar is dissolved. Cool.
- In a blender, blend together the cooled sugar water with the berries, water, lemon juice and mint leaves until well combined.
- Transfer the mixture to the refrigerator and let it cool completely, about 20 minutes.
- Pour into 1 large or 2 small bowls and enjoy.

Chapter 5 - Snacks Recipes

61) Wheat Crackers

Preparation time: 10 minutes. **Cooking time:** 20 minutes. **Servings: 4**

Ingredients:
- 1 3/4 cup of walnut flour
- 1 1/2 cups coconut flour
- 3/4 teaspoon sea salt

Directions:
- Set your oven to 350 degrees F.
- Mix the coconut flour, nut flour and salt in a bowl.
- Stir in vegetable oil and salt. Stir well until cooked through.
- Pour the dough onto a flat surface in a thin dish.

Ingredients:
- 1/3 vegetable oil
- 1 kitchen basket
- Sea salt for sprinkling

- Cut small squares out of the sheet.
- Arrange dough squares on a sheet of baking paper lined with parchment paper.
- Wet for 20 minutes until the light comes on.
- Serve.

62) Chips Potato

Preparation time: 10 mnutes. **Cooking time:** 5 minutes. **Servings: 4**

Ingredients:
- *1 tablespoon of vegetable oil*

Directions:
- Toss potato with oil and sea salt.
- Distribute the slices in a sandwich dish in a single row.

Ingredients:
- 1 potato, sliced paper thin Sea salt, to taste

- Bake for 5 minutes until golden brown.
- Serve.

63) Zucchini Pepper Chips

Preparation time: 10 minutes. **Cooking time:** 15 minutes. **Servings: 4**

Ingredients:
- 1 2/3 cups vegetable oil
- 1 teaspoon onion powder
- 1/2 teaspoon of black pepper

Directions:
- Mix the oil with all the spices in a bowl.
- Add the zucchini slices and mix well.
- Transfer the mixture into a container Zip lock and seal il.

172 Fat: 11.1g. Carbs: 19.9g. Protein: 13.5g. Fiber: 0.2g.

Ingredients:
- 3 tablespoons crushed red pepper flakes
- 2 zucchini, thinly sliced

- Refrigerate for 10 minutes.
- Spread the zuchini slices on a greased baking sheet.
- Bake for 15 minutes
- Serve.

64) Flat Bread

Preparation time: **Cooking Time:** 20 Minutes **Servings: 6**

Ingredients:
- 2 cups of Spelt Flour
- 2 teaspoons of Oregano
- 2 teaspoons of Onion powder
- 1/4 teaspoon of Cayenne

Directions:
- Add spelt flour and all grains to a bowl and mix well.
- Add the Grape Seed Oil and 1/2 cup of Spring Water and continue to mix.
- Try to form a thick ball. If it is too thick, add more Spring Water.
- Make a place to roll the mud and sprinkle it with flour.
- Knead the dough for about 5 minutes until it has become desired consistencyn.
- Divite the dough into 6 equal balls.

Ingredients:
- 2 teaspoons of basil
- 1 tablespoon of Pure Sea Salt
- 3/4 cup o of spring water
- 2 tablespoons of Grape Seed Oil
- Roll out each loaf in a circles container about 4 inches in diameter.
- Prepare a wooden skillet. Place one flatbred in the skillet and cook over medium heat.
- Flip the dish over for 2 to 3 minutes and work until dry. Small pieces of sugar paper should be placed on both sides.
- Keep looking at the upper body.
- Serve and enjoy your Flatbread!

65) Cracker Healthy

Preparation time: **Cooking time:** 30 minutes **Servings: 50 Crackers**

Ingredients:
- 1/2 cup of rye flour
- 1 cup of flour Spelt
- 2 teaspoons of Sesame Seed
- 1 teaspoon of Agave Syrup

Ingredients:
- 1 teaspoon of Pure Sea Salt
- 2 tablespoons of Grape Seed Oil
- 3/4 cup of Spring Water

Directions:
- Preheat our oven to 350 degrees Fahrenheit.
- Add all ingredients to a glass container and mix everything together.
- Make a ball of dough. If the dough is too thick, add more flour.
- Prepare a place to spread the dough and cover it with a piece of parchment paper.
- Degrease the container well with Grape Seed Oil and put the dart in it.
- RICE the slurry with a rolling pin, adding more flour so it doesn't fall apart.
- When your dough is ready, take a pastry cutter and insert it into the container. If you don't have a pastry cutter, you can use a cookie cutter.
- Arrange the squares on a kitchen basket and place them in the corner of a ech square using a fork of a skewer.
- Brush the plate with a little grain oil and sprinkle with a little pure sea salt, if needed.
- Bake for 12-15 minutes or until crackers are golden brown.
- Everything that was done was done with the help of another person.
- Serve and enjoy your Healthy Crackers!

66) Tortillas

Preparation time:. **Cooking Time:** 20 Minutes **Servings: 8**

Ingredients:
- 2 cups of flour Spelt
- 1 teaspoon of Pure Sea Salt

Ingredients:
- 1/2 cup of spring Water

Directions:
- In a food processor* blend the spelt flour with the pure salt. Blend for about 15 minutes.
- Blend, slowly add Grape seed oil until well distributed.
- Slowly add the soy water, stirring until a color forms.
- Prepare a piece of wallpaper and pour some parchment paper on it. Dust with a little flour.
- Process the nut for about 1 to 2 minutes until it reaches the right consistency.
- Pour dough into 8-inch pieces.
- Roll the sandwich into a very thin shape.
- Prepare a lunch box, cook one tortilla at a time in the microwave for about 30-60 minutes.
- Serve and enjoy your Tortillas!

67) Walnut Cheesecake Mango

Preparation time: **Cooking time:** 4 hours and 30 minutes **Servings: 8**

Ingredients:
- 2 cups of Brazil Nuts
- 5 to 6 Dates
- 1 tablespoon of Sea Moss Gel (check information)
- 1/4 cup o of agave syrup
- 1/4 teaspoon salt Pure Sea
- 2 tablespoons of Lime Juice
- 1 1/2 cups of Homemade Walnut Milk *

Ingredients:
Crust:
- 1 1/2 cups of quartered Dates 1/4 cup of Agave Syrup
- 1 1/2 cups of Coconut Flakes
- 1/4 teaspoon of Pure Sea Salt
- Toppings:
- Mango of Sliced
- Sliced strawberries

Directions:
- Place all crust ingredients in a processor and blend for 30 seconds.
- Prepare a baking sheet with a sheet of parchment and roll out the loose dough with butter.
- Place the Mango sliced across the crust and freeze for 10 minutes.
- Place all the glass pieces in a bowl until ready.
- Place the filling on top of the butter, wrap it with aluminum foil or a food container and let it rest for 3 to 4 hours in the refrigerator.
- Take out dalla baking form and garnish with toppings.
- Serve and enjoy our Mango Nut Cheesecake!

68) Blackberry Jam

Preparation time:

Cooking time: 4 hours and 30 minutes

Servings: 1 cup

Ingredients:
- 3/4 cup of Blackberries
- 1 tablespoon lime juice Key

Directions:
- Place blackberries in a medium saucepan and cook over low heat.
- Stir in blackberries until liquid is gone.
- Once you've picked the berries, use your blender to chop up the larger pieces. If you don't have a blender, put the mixture in an immersion blender, blend it well, and then return it to the oven.

Ingredients:
- 3 tablespoons of Agave Syrup
- ¼ cup of Sea Moss Gel + extra 2 tablespoons (check information)

- Add Sea Moss Gel, Key Lime Juice and Agave Syrup to the mixture. Cook over low heat and stir well until dry.
- Remove from heat and let sit for 10 minutes.
- Serve with pieces on flat bread.
- Enjoy your jam!

Helpful Hints: If you don't have Sea Moss Gel, you can omit it. However, the gel gives your skin a thinner, longer-lasting look. Blackberries have a natural pectin, which can have a similar effect. Store this Blackberry Jam in a glass jar with a lid in the refrigerator for 2 to 3 weeks. Do not store in extreme temperatures!

69) Blackberry Bars

Preparation time:

Cooking time: 1 hour 20 Minutes

Servings: 4

Ingredients:
- 3 Burro Banas or 4 Baby Banas
- 1 cup of Spelt Flour
- 2 cups of Quinoa Flakes
- 1/4 cup of Agave Syrup

Directions:
- Set the oven to 350 degrees Fahrenheit.
- Mash the bananas with a fork in a large bowl.
- Combine Agave Syrup and Grape Seed Oil to the puree and mix well.
- Add the Spelt flour and Quinoa flakes. Knead the dough until it becomes sticky to your finger.
- Prepare a 9x9-inch basket with a parchment lid.
- Take 2/3 of the dough and spread it with your fingers on the baking sheet parchment pan.

Ingredients:
- 1/4 teaspoon of Pure Sea Salt
- 1/2 cup of Grape Seed Oil
- 1 cup of prepared Blackberry Jam

- Spread Blackberry Jam over the dough.
- Crumble the rice and place it on the plate.
- Bake for 20 minutes.
- Remove from oven and let cool for 10-15 minutes.
- Cut into small pieces.
- Try and enjoy our Blackberry Bars!

70) SqUash Pie.

Preparation time:

Cooking time: 2 hours 30 Minutes

Servings: 6-8

Ingredients:
- 2 Butternut Squashes
- 1 1/4 cups of spelt flour
- 1/4 cup of dry sugar
- 1/4 cup of Agave Syrup
- 1 teaspoon of Allspice.

Directions:
- Rinse and peel butternut pumpkins.
- Cut them in half and use a spoon to de-sed.
- Cut the meat into one piece and place in a glass container.
- Cover the squash in Spring Water and boiltare for 20-25 minutes until coooked.
- Turn off the oven and mash the cooked squash.
- Add the date sugar, agave syrup, 1/8 pure sea salt, and homemade milk and mix everything together.
- Crust:
- Preheat the oven to 350 degrees Fahrenheit.
- In a bowl, add the spelt flour, 1/2 teaspoon of Pure Sea Salt, Spring Water, and Grape Seed Oil and mix.

Ingredients:
- 1 teaspoon of Pure Sea Salt
- 1/4 cup soy water
- 1/3 cup of fat seed oil
- 1/4 cup hemp seed milk Homemade *

- Reduce the rice into a loaf of bread. Add more water or flour if needed. Let stand for 5 minutes.
- Spread out Spelt Flour on a piece of parchment paper.
- Roll out on rolling pin, adding more flour to prevent sticking.
- Place the dough in a cake pan and bake for 10 minutes.
- Remove the butter from the oven, add the filling and bake for another 40 minutes.
- Remove the cake and let it rest for 30 minutes until cool.
- Serve enjoy your Squash Pie!

71) Walnut Milk Homemade

Preparation time: **Cooking time:** minimum 8 hours   **Servings:** 4 cups

Ingredients:
- 1 cup fresh walnuts
- 1/8 teaspoon of Pure Sea Salt

Ingredients:
- 3 cups of spring water + extra for soaking

Directions:
- Place the new Walnuts in a bag and fill it with three tablespoons of water.
- Take the Walnuts for an hour and a half.
- Drain and rinse nuts with warm water.
- Add the soaked walnuts, puree and three times the spring water to a blender.
- Mix well till smooth.
- Extend it if you need to.
- Enjoy your homemade nut milk!

Helpful Hints:

72) AqUafaba

Preparation time: **Cooking time:** 2 Hours 30 minutes   **Servings:** 2-4 cups

Ingredients:
- 1 bag of Garbanzo beans
- 1 teaspoon of Pure Sea Salt

Ingredients:
- 6 cups of Spring Water + extra for soaking

Directions:
- Place the chickpeas in a large pot, add the soy water and pure sea salt. Bring to a boil.
- Remove from heat and allow to soak 30 to 40 minutes.
- Strain the Garbanzo Beans and add 6 cups of water.
- Boil for 1 hour and 30 minutes on medium hat.
- Filter the Garbanzo beans. This filtered water is Aquafaba.
- Pour the Aquafaba into a glass jar with a lid and place in the refrigerator.
- After cooling, the Aquafaba becomes thicker. If it is too thick, boil for 10-20 mnutes.

73) Milk Homemade Hempsed

Preparation time: **Cooking time:** 2 hours   **Servings:** 2 cups

Ingredients:
- 2 tablespoons of Hemp Seeds
- 2 tablespoons of Agave Syrup

Ingredients:
- 1/8 teaspoon pure salt
- 2 cups of Spring Water Fruits (optional)*.

Directions:
- Place all ingredients, except fruit, in blender.
- Blend them for two minutes.
- Add fruits and resin for 30-50 minutes.
- Store milk in the refrigerator until aged.
- Enjoy your Homemade Hempsed Milk!

Helpful Hints:

74) Oil Spicy Infusion

Preparation time: **Cooking time:** 24 Hours   **Servings:** 1 cup

Ingredients:
- 1 tablespoon of crushed Cayenne Pepper

Ingredients:
- 3/4 cup of Grape Seed Oil

Directions:
- Fill a glass with a lid or bottle with grape oil.
- Add crushed Cayenne Pepper to the jar/bottle.
- Close and allow to cool for at least 24 hours.
- Add it to a dinner party and enjoy our Spicy Infuse oil!

Helpful Hints:

75) Italian Infused Oil

Preparation time: **Cooking time:** 24 hours **Servings:** 1 cup

Ingredients:
- 1 teaspoon of Oregano.
- 1 teaspoon of Basil

Directions:
- Fill a glass jar with a lid or container with grape oil.
- Mix the seasonings and add them to the rice and lettuce.

Ingredients:
- 1 pinch of salt Pure Sea
- 3/4 cup of Grape seed oil

- Shake and let the oil steep for at least 24 hours.
- Add it to a dish and enjoy your Infused Oil Italian!

76) Garlic Infused Oil

Preparation time: **Cooking time:** 24 hours **Servings:** 1 cup

Ingredients:
- 1/2 teaspoon of Dill
- 1/2 teaspoon of Ginger Powder
- 1 tablespoon of Onion Powder.

Directions:
- Fill a glass jar or squeeze bottle with grapeseed oil.
- Add the seasonings to the jar/bottle.

Ingredients:
- 1/2 teaspoon of Pure Sea Salt
- 3/4 cup of fat seed oil

- Close and let oil infuse for at least 24 hours.
- Add it to a dish and add your "Garlic". Infused Oil!

Helpful Hints:

77) Papaya Seeds Mango Dressing

Preparation time: **Cooking time:** 10 minutes **Servings:** 1/2 Cup

Ingredients:
- 1 cup of chopped Mango
- 1 teaspoon of Papaya Seeds Ground
- 1 teaspoon of Basil
- 1 teaspoon of Onion Powder

Directions:
- Prepare and place all ingredients into the mixture.
- Blend for one minute until smoth.

Ingredients:
- 1 teaspoon of Agave Syrup
- 2 tablespoons of lemon juice
- 1/4 cup of grape oil
- 1/4 teaspoon salt Pure Sea

- Add it to a dish and enjoy our Papaya Seed Mango Dress5ng!

Helpful Hints:

78) Blueberry Smoothie

Preparation time: 10 minutes **Cooking time:** **Servings:** 2

Ingredients:
- 2 cups of frozen blueberries
- 1 small banana

Directions:
- Place all ingredients in a high speed blender and pulse until creamy.

Ingredients:
- 1½ cups unsweetened almond milk
- ¼ cup ice cubes

- Pour the smoothie into two glasses and serve immediately.

Helpful Hints:

79) Raspberry And Tofu Smoothie

Preparation time: 10 minutes **Cooking time**: **Servings: 2**

Ingredients:
- 1½ cups of fresh raspberries
- 6 ounces of firm silken tofu, pressed and drained
- 4-5 drops of liquid stevia

Ingredients:
- 1 cup of coconut cream
- ¼ cup ice, crushed

Directions:
- Place all ingredients in a high speed blender and pulse until creamy.
- Pour the smoothie into two glasses and serve immediately.

80) Beet And Strawberry Smoothie

Preparation time: 10 minutes **Cooking time**: **Servings: 2**

Ingredients:
- 2 cups frozen strawberries, pitted and chopped
- ⅔ cup roasted and frozen beet, chopped
- 1 teaspoon fresh ginger, peeled and grated

Ingredients:
- 1 teaspoon fresh turmeric, peeled and grated
- ½ cup of fresh orange juice
- 1 cup unsweetened almond milk

Directions:
- Place all ingredients in a high speed blender and pulse until creamy.
- Pour the smoothie into two glasses and serve immediately.

Helpful Hints:

Chapter 6 - Dessert Recipes

81) Kiwi Smoothie

Preparation time: 10 minutes   **Cooking time**:   **Servings**: 2

Ingredients:
- 4 kiwis
- 2 small bananas, peeled
- 1½ cups unsweetened almond milk

Ingredients:
- 1-2 drops of liquid stevia
- ¼ cup ice cubes

Directions:
- Place all ingredients in a high speed blender and pulse until creamy.
- Pour the smoothie into two glasses and serve immediately.

Helpful Hints:

82) Pineapple And Carrot Smoothie

Preparation time: 10 minutes   **Cooking time**:   **Servings**: 2

Ingredients:
- 1 cup frozen pineapple
- 1 large ripe banana, peeled and sliced
- ½ tablespoon fresh ginger, peeled and chopped
- ¼ teaspoon ground turmeric

Ingredients:
- 1 cup unsweetened almond milk
- ½ cup fresh carrot juice
- 1 tablespoon fresh lemon juice

Directions:
- Place all ingredients in a high speed blender and pulse until creamy.
- Pour the smoothie into two glasses and serve immediately.

Helpful Hints:

83) Oatmeal And Orange Smoothie

Preparation time: 10 minutes   **Cooking time**:   **Servings**: 4

Ingredients:
- ⅔ cup of rolled oats
- 2 oranges, peeled, seeds removed and cut into sections
- 2 large bananas, peeled and sliced

Ingredients:
- 2 cups of unsweetened almond milk
- 1 cup ice cubes, crushed

Directions:
- Place all ingredients in a high speed blender and pulse until creamy.
- Pour the smoothie into four glasses and serve immediately.

Helpful Hints:

84) Pumpkin Smoothie

Preparation time: 10 minutes   **Cooking time**:   **Servings**: 2

Ingredients:
- 1 cup homemade pumpkin puree
- 1 medium banana, peeled and sliced
- 1 tablespoon maple syrup
- 1 teaspoon ground flax seeds

Ingredients:
- ½ teaspoon ground cinnamon
- ¼ teaspoon ground ginger
- 1½ cups unsweetened almond milk
- ¼ cup ice cubes

Directions:
- Place all ingredients in a high speed blender and pulse until creamy.
- Pour the smoothie into two glasses and serve immediately.

Nutrition: Calories

85) Red Fruit And Vegetable Smoothie

Preparation time: 10 minutes **Cooking time**: **Servings: 2**

Ingredients:
- ½ cup fresh raspberries
- ½ cup fresh strawberries
- ½ red bell pepper, seeded and chopped
- ½ cup red cabbage, chopped

Directions:
- Place all ingredients in a high speed blender and pulse until creamy.

Ingredients:
- 1 small tomato
- 1 cup of water
- ½ cup of ice cubes
- Pour the smoothie into two glasses and serve immediately.

86) Kale Smoothie

Preparation time: 10 minutes **Cooking time**: **Servings: 2**

Ingredients:
- 3 fresh cabbage stalks, cut and chopped
- 1-2 celery stalks, chopped
- ½ avocado, peeled, pitted and chopped

Directions:
- Place all ingredients in a high speed blender and pulse until creamy.

Ingredients:
- ½ inch ginger root, chopped
- ½ inch turmeric root, chopped
- 2 cups of coconut milk
- Pour the smoothie into two glasses and serve immediately.

87) Green Tofu Smoothie

Preparation time: 10 minutes **Cooking time**: **Servings: 2**

Ingredients:
- 1½ cups cucumber, peeled and coarsely chopped
- 3 cups fresh spinach
- 2 cups of frozen broccoli
- ½ cup silken tofu, drained and pressed

Directions:
- Place all ingredients in a high speed blender and pulse until creamy.

Ingredients:
- 1 tablespoon fresh lime juice
- 4-5 drops of liquid stevia
- 1 cup unsweetened almond milk
- ½ cup ice, crushed
- Pour the smoothie into two glasses and serve immediately.

88) Grape And Chard Smoothie

Preparation time: 10 minutes **Cooking time**: **Servings: 2**

Ingredients:
- 2 cups of green grapes without seeds
- 2 cups fresh beets, cut and chopped
- 2 tablespoons of maple syrup

Directions:
- Place all ingredients in a high speed blender and pulse until creamy.

Ingredients:
- 1 teaspoon fresh lemon juice
- 1½ cups of water
- 4 ice cubes
- Pour the smoothie into two glasses and serve immediately.

89) Matcha Smoothie

Preparation time: 10 minutes   **Cooking time**:   **Servings: 2**

Ingredients:
- 2 tablespoons of chia seeds
- 2 teaspoons of matcha green tea powder
- ½ teaspoon fresh lemon juice
- ½ teaspoon xanthan gum

Directions:
- Place all ingredients in a high speed blender and pulse until creamy.

Ingredients:
- 8-10 drops of liquid stevia
- 4 tablespoons of coconut cream
- 1½ cups unsweetened almond milk
- ¼ cup ice cubes
- Pour the smoothie into two glasses and serve immediately.

90) Banana Smoothie

Preparation time: 10 minutes   **Cooking time**:   **Servings: 2**

Ingredients:
- 2 cups of cooled unsweetened almond milk
- 1 large frozen banana, peeled and sliced

Directions:
- Place all ingredients in a high speed blender and pulse until creamy.

Ingredients:
- 1 tablespoon almonds, chopped
- 1 teaspoon of organic vanilla extract
- Pour the smoothie into two glasses and serve immediately.

91) Strawberry Smoothie

Preparation time: 10 minutes   **Cooking time**:   **Servings: 2**

Ingredients:
- 2 cups of cooled unsweetened almond milk
- 1½ cups of frozen strawberries

Directions:
- Add all ingredients to a high speed blender and pulse until smooth.

Ingredients:
- 1 banana, peeled and sliced
- ¼ teaspoon of organic vanilla extract
- Pour the smoothie into two glasses and serve immediately.

92) Raspberry And Tofu Smoothie

Preparation time: 15 minutes   **Cooking time**:   **Servings: 2**

Ingredients:
- 1½ cups of fresh raspberries
- 6 ounces of firm silken tofu, drained
- 1/8 teaspoon of coconut extract

Directions:
- Add all ingredients to a high speed blender and pulse until smooth.

Ingredients:
- 1 teaspoon of stevia powder
- 1½ cups unsweetened almond milk
- ¼ cup ice cubes, crushed
- Pour the smoothie into two glasses and serve immediately.

93) Mango Smoothie

Preparation time: 10 minutes   **Cooking time:**   **Servings:** 2

Ingredients:
- 2 cups frozen mango, peeled, pitted and chopped
- ¼ cup almond butter
- Pinch of ground turmeric
- 2 tablespoons fresh lemon juice
- 1¼ cup unsweetened almond milk
- ¼ cup ice cubes

Directions:
- Add all ingredients to a high speed blender and pulse until smooth.
- Pour the smoothie into two glasses and serve immediately.

94) Pineapple Smoothie

Preparation time: 10 minutes   **Cooking time:**   **Servings:** 2

Ingredients:
- 2 cups pineapple, chopped
- ½ teaspoon fresh ginger, peeled and chopped
- ½ teaspoon ground turmeric
- 1 teaspoon of natural immune support supplement*.
- 1 teaspoon of chia seeds
- 1½ cups of cold green tea
- ½ cup ice, crushed

Directions:
- Add all ingredients to a high speed blender and pulse until smooth.
- Pour the smoothie into two glasses and serve immediately.

95) Cabbage And Pineapple Smoothie

Preparation time: 15 minutes   **Cooking time:**   **Servings:** 2

Ingredients:
- 1½ cups fresh cabbage, chopped and shredded
- 1 frozen banana, peeled and chopped
- ½ cup of fresh pineapple chunks
- 1 cup unsweetened coconut milk
- ½ cup of fresh orange juice
- ½ cup of ice

Directions:
- Add all ingredients to a high speed blender and pulse until smooth.
- Pour the smoothie into two glasses and serve immediately.

96) Green Vegetable Smoothie

Preparation time: 15 minutes   **Cooking time:**   **Servings:** 2

Ingredients:
- 1 medium avocado, peeled, pitted and chopped
- 1 large cucumber, peeled and chopped
- 2 fresh tomatoes, chopped
- 1 small green bell pepper, seeded and chopped
- 1 cup fresh spinach, torn
- 2 tablespoons fresh lime juice
- 2 tablespoons of homemade vegetable broth
- 1 cup of alkaline water

Directions:
- Add all ingredients to a high speed blender and pulse until smooth.
- Pour smoothie into glasses and serve immediately.

97) Avocado And Spinach Smoothie

Preparation time: 10 minutes   **Cooking time**:   **Servings**: 2

Ingredients:
- 2 cups of fresh spinach
- ½ avocado, peeled, pitted and chopped
- 4-6 drops of liquid stevia

Directions:
- Add all ingredients to a high speed blender and pulse until smooth.

Ingredients:
- ½ teaspoon ground cinnamon
- 1 tablespoon of hemp seeds
- 2 cups of cooled alkaline water
- Pour the smoothie into two glasses and serve immediately.

98) Cucumber Smoothie

Preparation time: 15 minutes   **Cooking time**:   **Servings**: 2

Ingredients:
- 1 small cucumber, peeled and chopped
- 2 cups fresh mixed greens (spinach, kale, chard), chopped and shredded
- ½ cup of lettuce, torn
- ¼ cup fresh parsley leaves
- ¼ cup fresh mint leaves

Directions:
- Add all ingredients to a high speed blender and pulse until smooth.

Ingredients:
- 2-3 drops of liquid stevia
- 1 teaspoon fresh lemon juice
- 1½ cups of filtered water
- ¼ cup ice cubes
- Pour the smoothie into two glasses and serve immediately.

99) Apple And Ginger Smoothie

Preparation time: 10 minutes   **Cooking time**: 0 minutes   **Servings**: 1

Ingredients:
- 1 apple, peeled and diced
- ¾ cup (6 ounces) of coconut yogurt

Directions:
- Add all ingredients to a blender.
- Blend well until smooth.

Ingredients:
- ½ teaspoon of ginger, freshly grated
- Refrigerate for 2 to 3 hours.
- Serve.

100) Green Tea Blueberry Smoothie

Preparation time: 10 minutes   **Cooking time**: 5 minutes   **Servings**: 1

Ingredients:
- 3 tablespoons of alkaline water
- 1 green tea bag
- 1 ½ cups fresh blueberries

Directions:
- Boil 3 tablespoons of water in a small saucepan and transfer to a cup.
- Dip the tea bag into the cup and let it sit for 4 to 5 minutes.
- Discard the tea bag and
- Transfer the green tea to a blender

Ingredients:
- 1 pear, peeled, stoned and diced
- ¾ cup of almond milk
- Add all other ingredients to blender.
- Blend well until smooth.
- Serve with fresh blueberries.

Chapter 7 - Dr. Lewis's Meal Plan Project

Day 1

18)	Amaranth porridge
24)	Crockpot Summer Vegetables
55)	Watermelon and jalapeno gazpacho
62)	Chips potato
55)	Watermelon and jalapeno gazpacho

Day 2

9)	Avocado Toast
23)	Roasted vegetables
52)	Coconut and cashew soup with tarragon
65)	Cracker Healthy
58)	Cauliflower and roasted garlic soup

Day 3

13)	Alkaline Blueberry Spelt Pancakes
28)	Rainbow salad with Meyer lemon dressing
48)	Chayote mushroom and hemp milk stew
67)	Walnut cheesecake Mango
64)	Flat bread

Day 4

15)	Meal of crispy quinoa
32)	Rice with sesame and ginger
59)	Carrot and potato stew with herbs
72)	Aquafaba
68)	Blackberry Jam

Day 5

4)	Banana porridge
33)	Macaroni and 'Cheese
43)	Green zucchini soup
77)	Papaya Seeds Mango Dressing
88)	Grape and chard smoothie

Day 6

7)	Zucchini fritters
36)	Jamaican Jerk Patties
45)	Pumpkin soup with basil
79)	Raspberry and tofu smoothie
79)	Raspberry and tofu smoothie

Day 7

1)	Baked grapefruit
38)	Mushroom burgers Portobello
41)	Cabbage, soursop and zucchini soup
91)	Strawberry Smoothie
99)	Apple and Ginger Smoothie

Chapter 8 - Conclusion

I hope this book can lead you to your goals, keeping your desire to keep going high, without making you lose sight of the outcome

This book series is designed to help women, men, athletes and sportsmen, people immersed in work with little free time, etc.

If you recognize yourself in one of these categories or someone you know has decided to take the same path as you,

You'll find the other books in the series in your trusted bookstore, guaranteed!

Big hugs from Dr. Grace!

Alkaline Diet Cookbook on a Budget

Dr. Lewis's Meal Plan Project | 100 Affordable, Easy-To-Prepare Recipes to Kickstart Your Long-Term Transformation Path Without Emptying Your Wallet

By Grace Lewis

Chapter 1 - Introduction

Starting a diet path may be the hardest choice to make, but it will be the best choice you will ever make in your life.

The alkaline diet can help you embark on your path of change much more easily than other diet paths.

In most cases an individual is inclined to think that rigidly adhering to a diet plan will lead him or her to spend much more money than the family budget normally allows.

In this book I have put together all my best low budget recipes, accompanied by an eating plan to experience the benefits of the alkaline diet right away.

The important thing is to get started, without thinking about your wallet.

I wish you a speedy achievement of your goals.

Here's to your success!

Grace

Chapter 2 -   Breakfast Recipes

1) Mile Porridge

Preparation time: 10 minutes. **Cooking time**: 20 minutes. **Servings**: 2

Ingredients:
- Sea salt
- 1 tbsp. finely chopped coconuts.
- 1/2 cup unsweetened coconut milk

Directions:
- Sauté the millet in a non-stick skillet for about 3 minutes.
- Add salt and water, then stir.
- Allow the meal to rest and reduce the amount of salt.

Nutrition: Calories

Ingredients:
- 1/2 cup millet rinsed and millet draned
- 1-1/2 cups water alkaline
- 3 Drops liquid stevia.
- Cook for about 15 minutes, then add remaining ingredients. Stylize.
- Cook the apple for an additional 4 minutes.
- Serve the meal with a garnish of hazelnuts chopped.

2) Jackfruit Fry vegetable

Preparation time: 5 minutes. **Cooking time**: 5 minutes. **Servings**: 6

Ingredients:
- 2 onions small finely chopped
- 2 cups tomatoes chopped cherry finely
- 1/8 tablespoon of cassava butter
- 1 tablespoon olive oil

Directions:
- In a fat skillet, saute onions and bell peppers for about 5 minutes.
- Add tomatoes and stir.
- Coook for 2 minutes.

Nutrition: Calories

Ingredients:
- 2 seeded and chopped red bell peppers
- 3 cups firm jackfruit with seeds and chopped
- 1/8 teaspoon cayenne pepper
- 2 tbsps. Chopped fresh basil leaves Salt
- Then add the juice, pepper, salt and turmeric.
- Bake for about 8 minutes.
- Garnish the meal with basil leaves.
- Serve hot.

3) Zucchini Pancakes

Preparation time: 15 minutes. **Cooking time**: 8 minutes. **Servings**: 8

Ingredients:
- 12 tablespoons of alkaline water
- 6 great zucchini grateds
- Sea salt
- 4 tbsp of Flax Seeds chopped

Directions:
- In a bowl, mix together the water and flax and then set aside.
- Place our food in a large non-stick container and then place it in a cooking container.
- Add the glass of milk, the glass of wine, and the glass of pumpkin.
- Coook for 3 minutes then transfer the zucchini into a large boge.

Nutrition: Calories

Ingredients:
- 2 tsps. Olive oil
- 2 jalapeño peppers finely chopped
- 1/2 cup finely chopped scallions
- Add the flax and scallion mixture and then mix everything together.
- Preheat a grill and then grease it well with oil.
- Pour 1/4 zuchini mixture into a griddle and bake for 3 minutes.
- Flip the side carefully then coook for 2 more minutes.
- Repeat the procedure with the rest of the mass in random order.
- Serve.

4) Squash Hash

Preparation time: 2 mnutes. **Cooking time**: 10 minutes. **Servings**: 2

Ingredients:
- 1 tsp. onion powder.
- 1/2 cup finely chopped onion

Directions:
- By using paper towels, you can get extra moisture from the spaghetti squash.
- Place the squash in a bowl, then add the salt, onion and onion powder.
- Stir well to mix everything together.
- Spray a non-stick cooking skillet with coooking spray that place il over moderate heat.

Ingredients:
- 2 cups of spaghetti squash
- 1/2 teaspoon of sea salt
- Add the spaghetti squash.
- Coook the squash for 5 minutes.
- Smash the browns with a spatula.
- Coook formatis of 5 minutes until the desired crispness is reached.
- Serve.

5) Hemp Seed Porridge

Preparation time: 5 minutes. **Cooking time:** 5 minutes. **Servings: 6**

Ingredients:
- ✓ 3 cups cooked hemp sed
- ✓ 1 packet Stevia

Directions:
- ❖ In a bowl, mix the milk and nut milk for about 5 minutes.
- ❖ Remove the pan from the heat and add the stevia. Stylize.

Ingredients:
- ✓ 1 cup coco of walnut milk

- ❖ Serve in 6 bowls.
- ❖ Enjoy.

Nutrition: Calories

6) Veggie Medley

Preparation time: 5 mnutes. **Cooking time:** 10 minutes. **Servings: 2**

Ingredients:
- ✓ 1 seed and 1 bacon
- ✓ 1/2 cup lime juice
- ✓ 2 tablespoons of fresh cilantro
- ✓ 1/2 tsp. cumin
- ✓ 1 teaspoon of sea salt
- ✓ 1 wooden jacket

Directions:
- ❖ Spray some paint with stick pan with cooking spray and then put it all over your body.
- ❖ Add the butter, tomatoes, chili, grapes, pumpkin, peanut butter and mushroms.

Ingredients:
- ✓ 1/2 cup zucchini
- ✓ 1 cup halved cherry tomatoes
- ✓ 1/2 cup sliced mushrooms
- ✓ 1 cup coooked broccoli florets
- ✓ 1 sweet onion chopped

- ❖ Cook for about 7 minutes as you stir from time to time.
- ❖ Add the cumin and caraway and then the pepper.
- ❖ Cook for an additional 3 minutes, stirring.
- ❖ Heat the pan off the heat and add the lime juice.
- ❖ Serve.

Nutrition: Calories

7) Pumpkin Spice Quinoa

Preparation time: 10 minutes. **Cooking time:** 0 minutes. **Servings: 2**

Ingredients:
- ✓ 1 cup of cooked quinoa
- ✓ 1 cup unsweetened coconut milk
- ✓ 1 large mashed banana

Directions:
- ❖ In a container, mix all ingredients together.
- ❖ Close the lid and then close the container so that it mixes.

Ingredients:
- ✓ 1/4 cup pumpkin pureee
- ✓ 1 tsp. pumpkin spice
- ✓ 2 teaspoons of chia seds

- ❖ Refrigerate overnight.
- ❖ Serve.

Nutrition: Calories

8) Coconut pulp Coookies

Preparation time: 5 minutes. **Cooking time:** 10 hours. **Servings: 4**

Ingredients:
- ✓ 3 cups coconut pulp
- ✓ 1 Granny Smith apple
- ✓ 1-2 teaspoon cinnamon

Directions:
- ❖ Blend the coconut with the remaining ingredients in a processor food processor.
- ❖ Make many cookies with this mixture.
- ❖ Arrange them on a kitchen table, lined with parchment.

Ingredients:
- ✓ 2-3 tablespoons of raw honey
- ✓ 1/4 cup coco walnut flakes

- ❖ Place the dough in a food grade oven for 6-10 hours at 115 degrees Fahrenheit.
- ❖ Serve.

Nutrition: Calories 240 Fat: 22.5g. Carbohydrates: 17.3g. Protein: 14.9g. Fiber: 0g.

9) Avocado Pudding

Preparation time: 10 minutes   **Cooking time**: 0 minutes   **Servings**: 2

Ingredients:
- 2 avocados
- 3/4-1 cup coconut milk
- 1/3-1/2 cup of raw cacao powder

Directions:
- Mix all ingredients together in a blender.

Ingredients:
- 1 teaspoon 100% pure organic vanilla (optional)
- 2-4 tablespoons of date sugar

- Refrigerate for 4 hours in a container.
- Serve.

Nutrition: Calories 609 Fats: 50.5g. Carbs: 9.9g. Protein: 29.3g. Fiber: 1.5g.

10) Coconut Raisins cooookies

Preparation time: 10 minutes.   **Cooking time**: 10 minutes.   **Servings**: 4

Ingredients:
- 1 1/4 cups of coconut flour 1 cup of nut flour
- 1 teaspoon baking soda
- 1/2 Celtic teaspoon sea salt
- 1 button for peanuts cup
- 1 cup coconut date sugar

Directions:
- Turn on the oven to 357 degrees F.
- Mix the flour with the salt and baking soda.
- Flatten with sugar until started and then stirs in the nut milk and vinavilla.

Ingredients:
- 2 teaspoons of vanilla
- ¼ cup coconut milk
- 3/4 cup organic raisins
- 3/4 cup coconut chips or flakes

- Mix well, then place in a powder container. Stir until fine.
- Add all remaining ingredients.
- Make small cooookies out this dough.
- Arrange the cookies on a baking sheet.
- Bake for 10 minutes until set.

Nutrition: Calories 237 Fat: 19.8g. Carbs: 55.1g. Protein: 17.8g. Fiber: 0.9g.

11) Cracker Pumpkin Spice

Preparation time: 10 minutes.   **Cooking time**: 1 hour.   **Servings**: 6

Ingredients:
- 1/3 cup coco walnut flour
- 2 tablespoons pumpkin pie spice
- ¾ cup sunflower seds
- ¾ cup flaxseed
- 1/3 cup sesame seeds

Directions:
- Heat our oven to 300 degrees F. Combine all ingredients in a bowl.
- Add the salt and oil to the mixture and mix well.
- Allow the dough to rest for 2 to 3 minutes.

Ingredients:
- 1 tablespoon gron psyllium husk powder
- 1 teaspoon sea salt
- 3 tablespoons coco walnut oil, melted
- 1 1/3 cups water

- Roll out the dough on a cookie sheet lined with parchment paper.
- Bake for 30 minutes.
- Reduce the amount of food to 30 m weight and let it rest for another 30 m.
- Crush the bread into small pieces. Serve

Nutrition: Calories 248 Fat: 15.7g. Carbs: 0.4g. Protein: 24.9g. Fiber: 0g.

12) Spicy Toasted nuts

Preparation time: 10 minutes.   **Cooking time**: 15 minutes.   **Servings**: 4

Ingredients:
- 8 ounces of pecans or coconuts or walnuts
- 1 teaspoon of sea salt
- 1 tablespoon olive oil or coconut oil

Directions:
- Add all ingredients to an oven. Brown nuts until golden brown.

Ingredients:
- 1 teaspoon of ground cumin
- 1 teaspoon of paprika powder or chili powder

- Serve and enjoy.

Nutrition: Calories 287 Fat: 29.5g. Carbohydrates: 5.9g. Protein: 4.2g. Fiber: 4.3g.

13) Wheat Crackers

Preparation time: 10 minutes.   **Cooking time:** 20 minutes.   **Servings:** 4

Ingredients:
- 1 3/4 cup of walnut flour
- 1 1/2 cups coconut flour
- 3/4 teaspoon sea salt

Ingredients:
- 1/3 vegetable oil
- 1 kitchen basket
- Sea salt for sprinkling

Directions:
- Set your oven to 350 degrees F.
- Mix the coconut flour, nut flour and salt in a bowl.
- Stir in vegetable oil and salt. Stir well until cooked through.
- Pour the dough onto a flat surface in a thin dish.
- Cut small squares out of the sheet.
- Arrange dough squares on a sheet of baking paper lined with parchment paper.
- Wet for 20 minutes until the light comes on.
- Serve.

Nutrition: Calories 64 Fat: 9.2g. Carbs: 9.2g. Protein: 1.5g. Fiber: 0.9g.

14) Chips potato

Preparation time: 10 mnutes.   **Cooking time:** 5 minutes.   **Servings:** 4

Ingredients:
- 1 tablespoon of vegetable oil

Ingredients:
- 1 potato, sliced paper thin Sea salt, to taste

Directions:
- Toss potato with oil and sea salt.
- Distribute the slices in a sandwich dish in a single row.
- Bake for 5 minutes until golden brown.
- Serve.

Nutrition: Calories 80 Fat: 3.5g. Carbohydrates: 11.6g. Protein: 1.2g.

15) Zucchini Pepper Chips

Preparation time: 10 minutes.   **Cooking time:** 15 minutes.   **Servings:** 4

Ingredients:
- 1 2/3 cups vegetable oil
- 1 teaspoon onion powder
- 1/2 teaspoon of black pepper

Ingredients:
- 3 tablespoons crushed red pepper flakes
- 2 zucchini, thinly sliced

Directions:
- Mix the oil with all the spices in a bowl.
- Add the zucchini slices and mix well.
- Transfer the mixture into a container Zip lock and seal il.
- Refrigerate for 10 minutes.
- Spread the zuchini slices on a greased baking sheet.
- Bake for 15 minutes
- Serve.

Nutrition: Calories 172 Fat: 11.1g. Carbs: 19.9g. Protein: 13.5g. Fiber: 0.2g.

16) Flat bread

Preparation time: **Cooking Time:** 20 Minutes   **Servings:** 6

Ingredients:
- 2 cups of Spelt Flour
- 2 teaspoons of Oregano
- 2 teaspoons of Onion powder
- 1/4 teaspoon of Cayenne

Ingredients:
- 2 teaspoons of basil
- 1 tablespoon of Pure Sea Salt
- 3/4 cup o of spring water
- 2 tablespoons of Grape Seed Oil

Directions:
- Add spelt flour and all grains to a bowl and mix well.
- Add the Grape Seed Oil and 1/2 cup of Spring Water and continue to mix.
- Try to form a thick ball. If it is too thick, add more Spring Water.
- Make a place to roll the mud and sprinkle it with flour.
- Knead the dough for about 5 minutes until it has become desired consistencyn.
- Divite the dough into 6 equal balls.
- Roll out each loaf in a circles container about 4 inches in diameter.
- Prepare a wooden skillet. Place one flatbred in the skillet and oook over medium heat.
- Flip the dish over for 2 to 3 minutes and work until dry. Small pieces of sugar paper should be placed on both sides.
- Keep looking at the upper body.
- Serve and enjoy your Flatbread!

Nutrition: Calories

17) Cracker Healthy

Preparation time: **Cooking time:** 30 minutes **Servings:** 50 Crackers

Ingredients:
- 1/2 cup of rye flour
- 1 cup of flour Spelt
- 2 teaspoons of Sesame Seed
- 1 teaspoon of Agave Syrup

Directions:
- Preheat our oven to 350 degrees Fahrenheit.
- Add all ingredients to a glass container and mix everything together.
- Make a ball of dough. If the dough is too thick, add more flour.
- Prepare a place to spread the dough and cover it with a piece of parchment paper.
- Degrease the container well with Grape Seed Oil and put the dart in it.
- RICE the slurry with a rolling pin, adding more flour so it doesn't fall apart.

Ingredients:
- 1 teaspoon of Pure Sea Salt
- 2 tablespoons of Grape Seed Oil
- 3/4 cup of Spring Water

- When your dough is ready, take a pastry cutter and insert it into the container. If you don't have a pastry cutter, you can use a cookie cutter.
- Arrange the squares on a kitchen basket and place them in the corner of a ech square using a fork of a skewer.
- Brush the plate with a little grain oil and sprinkle with a little pure sea salt, if needed.
- Bake for 12-15 minutes or until crackers are golden brown.
- Everything that was done was done with the help of another person.
- Serve and enjoy your Healthy Crackers!

Nutrition: Calories

Helpful Hints: You can add any seasonings from the Doctor Sebi's food list according to your desire. You can make crackers with our tomato sauce, avocado sauce or cheese. Sauce.

18) Tortillas

Preparation time:. **Cooking Time:** 20 Minutes **Servings:** 8

Ingredients:
- 2 cups of flour Spelt
- 1 teaspoon of Pure Sea Salt

Directions:
- In a food processor* blend the spelt flour with the pure salt. Blend for about 15 minutes.
- Blend, slowly add Grape seed oil until well distributed.
- Slowly add the soy water, stirring until a color forms.
- Prepare a piece of wallpaper and pour some parchment paper on it. Dust with a little flour.

Ingredients:
- 1/2 cup of spring Water

- Process the nut for about 1 to 2 minutes until it reaches the right consistency.
- Pour dough into 8-inch pieces.
- Roll the sandwich into a very thin shape.
- Prepare a lunch box, cook one tortilla at a time in the microwave for about 30-60 minutes.
- Serve and enjoy your Tortillas!

Nutrition: Calories

Helpful Hints: If you don't have a refrigerator, you can use a mixer or blender. However, you will have a better result with a food as you have nothing to do with. You can serve the Tortillas with our Sweet Butter Sauce, Avocado Sauce or Cheese. Sauce.

19) Pink Smoothie

Preparation time: 10 minutes **Cooking time:** 0 minutes **Servings:** 1

Ingredients:
- 1 peach, core and peel
- 6 ripe strawberries

Directions:
- Add all ingredients to a blender.

Ingredients:
- 1 cup of almond milk

- Blend well until smooth.
- Serve with your favorite berries

Nutrition: Calories

20) Green Apple Smoothie

Preparation time: 10 minutes **Cooking time:** 0 minutes **Servings:** 1

Ingredients:
- 1 peach, peeled and pitted
- 1 green apple, peeled and cored

Directions:
- Add all ingredients to a blender.

Ingredients:
- 1 cup of alkaline water

- Blend well until smooth.
- Serve with apple slices.

Chapter 3 - Lunch Recipes

21) Roasted artichoke salad

Preparation time: Cooking time: Servings: 2

Ingredients:
- Paprika, pinch
- Garlic powder, a pinch
- Pepper, pinch
- Sea salt, a pinch
- Avocado oil, 1 tablespoon
- Drained artichoke hearts, 14 ounces
- Mixed salad, 2-4 c.

Directions:
- Start by setting the oven to 425. Place parchment on a baking sheet.
- Cut off the tips of the artichokes and then cut the hearts in half. Rub them with a little oil.
- Stir in paprika, garlic, pepper and salt. Arrange artichokes on baking sheet and sprinkle with seasoning mixture. Stir to coat.

Ingredients:
- Seasoning -
- Pepper, pinch
- Sea salt, a pinch
- Shallot diced
- Brown rice sweetener, 1 tablespoon
- Sesame seeds, 1 tablespoon
- Apple vinegar, 2 tablespoons
- Avocado oil, 2 tablespoons
- Roast them for 30 minutes, tossing again halfway through the cooking time.
- While the artichokes are roasting, whisk together the pepper, salt, shallots, brown rice syrup, sesame seeds, vinegar and avocado oil. Make sure everything is well blended. Adjust the flavors as needed.
- To assemble the salad, toss the salad with the artichokes and then pour in the dressing. Divide between two plates and enjoy.

Nutrition: Calories

22) Artichoke pie

Preparation time: Cooking time: Servings: 4

Ingredients:
- Sliced shallot
- EVOO
- Pepper

Directions:
- Pour cold water into a bowl.
- Place the sliced artichokes in the water and let them rest.
- Rinse well and pat dry with paper towels.
- Place a skillet over medium heat and heat a little EVOO.

Ingredients:
- Halls
- Brussels sprouts thinly sliced, 6
- Sliced mushrooms, 4
- Add the artichokes and Brussels sprouts. Cook for four minutes.
- Sprinkle with pepper and salt.
- Serve with a drizzle of olive oil and sprinkle with sliced scallions

Nutrition: Calories

23) Vegetable fritters

Preparation time: Cooking time: Servings: 2

Ingredients:
- Kitchen spray
- Water, .25 c.
- Garlic powder, .5 tsp
- Salt, 1 teaspoon
- Almond flour, .25 c.

Directions:
- Place the scallions, almond flour, yellow squash, zucchini, carrot, garlic powder and salt in a food processor.
- Pulse until everything is completely mixed.
- Add just enough water to make sure the dough is moist and thick.

Ingredients:
- Shallots, 4
- Grated onion, .5
- Chopped yellow pumpkin, 1
- Peeled and chopped carrot, 1
- Chopped zucchini, 1
- Place a large skillet over standard heat and spray with prep spray.
- When the oil is heated, use an ice cream scoop and add the mixture to the pan. Cook for three minutes per side.
- Use the back of the ice cream scoop to spread the mixture.

Nutrition: Calories

24) Mint and lime salad

Preparation time: Cooking time: Servings: 4

Ingredients:
- Lemon juice, 2 tablespoons
- Chopped mint, 2 tablespoons
- Strawberries, .25 c.
- Diced peaches, .25 c.
- Mandarin segments, .25 c.

Directions:
- Place all the fruit in a bowl. Add the mint and lemon juice.

Nutrition: Calories

Ingredients:
- Chopped melon pieces, .25 c.
- Pieces of honeydew chunks, .25 c.
- Watermelon chunks, .25 c.
- Diced apple, .25 c.
- Grapes, .25 c.
- Mix well and cover.
- Refrigerate and chill overnight.

25) Zucchini salad

Preparation time: Cooking time: Servings: 2

Ingredients:
- Fresh herbs of your choice, 1 teaspoon
- Pepper
- Halls
- EVOO, 2 tablespoons
- Juice of 0,5 lemons

Directions:
- Wash all the vegetables and set aside.
- Cut off the ends of the zucchini. Cut in half lengthwise and then slice into half moons.
- Dice the tomatoes.
- Cut the bell bell pepper in half, clean the ribs and seeds and slice each half.

Nutrition: Calories

Ingredients:
- Chopped garlic, 1 clove
- Sliced onion, 1
- Diced tomato, 2
- Red bell pepper, 1
- Sliced zucchini, 1
- Cut off top and bottom of onion and remove outer skin. Thinly slice into rings.
- Add all prepared vegetables to a bowl.
- In a separate bowl, add pepper, salt, herbs, olive oil, garlic and lemon juice. Mix well to combine.
- Pour over vegetables and stir to coat.

26) Fried tofu

Preparation time: Cooking time: Portions:

Ingredients:
- Fresh herbs
- Ginger, .25 tablespoons
- Curry powder, .5 tablespoons
- Pepper
- Halls
- EVOO, 2 tablespoons
- Coconut milk, 1.5 c.
- Chopped green beans, .5 lb.

Directions:
- Place a saucepan over medium heat, heat the oil. Add the tofu and cook about three minutes.
- Add the zucchini, beans and peppers. Sauté for an additional three minutes.

Nutrition: Calories

Ingredients:
- Diced bell pepper - green, bell, 1 piece
- Diced red bell pepper, bell, 1 piece
- Diced tomatoes, 3
- Chopped zucchini, 3
- Diced firm tofu, 1 lb.

- Add the tomatoes and coconut milk and mix well. Allow to simmer for a bit longer.
- Season with herbs, curry powder, pepper, salt and ginger.
- Serve with wild rice.

27) Potato and pumpkin meatballs

Preparation time: Cooking time: Servings: 2

Ingredients:
- EVOO
- Pepper
- Halls
- Chopped parsley, 3 tablespoons

Directions:
- Peel the potatoes and squash. Cut them into large pieces.
- Place in a food processor and process until small pieces but not mush.
- Add the water and soy flour to a bowl. Stir well.
- Remove the squash and potato from the food processor and place them in another bowl.

Ingredients:
- Water, 4 tablespoons
- Soybean flour, 2.5 ounces
- Potatoes, 1 lb.
- Pumpkin, 1 lb.
- Pour over flour mixture and mix well.
- Season with pepper, parsley and salt.
- Place a skillet over medium heat and heat a little EVOO.
- Turn the potato and pumpkin mixture into meatballs. Place the prepared patties in the skillet and fry for three minutes per side.

Nutrition: Calories

28) Italian soffritto

Preparation time: Cooking time: Servings: 2

Ingredients:
- Water, .5 c
- Pepper
- Curry powder, .5 teaspoons
- Oregano plant, 1 teaspoon
- Parsley, one tablespoon
- Sodium chloride, 1 teaspoon

Directions:
- Take a frying pan and heat the olive oil.
- Place the onions in the skillet and cook until soft.
- Add the zucchini and cook an additional four minutes. Pour the water into the pan and put a lid on.
- Lower the heat and simmer for ten minutes.

Ingredients:
- Grated Cheddar, 1 tablespoon
- EVOO, 2 tablespoons
- Diced tomatoes, 2
- Zucchini flakes, 1
- Diced onion, 2
- Leeks in flakes, 2
- Carefully remove the lid and add the tomatoes. Season with curry powder and pepper. Replace the lid and cook another ten minutes.
- When cooked, taste and adjust seasonings if necessary.
- Sprinkle with cheese and serve with bread, if your diet permits.

Nutrition: Calories

29) Southern Salad

Preparation time: Cooking time: Servings: 4

Ingredients:
- Sauce, .5 c.
- Cilantro, .5 c.
- Chopped almonds, .25 c.
- Diced avocado, 1

Directions:
- Place each content in a large bowl and mix well.

Ingredients:
- Halved cherry tomatoes, 1 c.
- Sprouted black beans, .5 c.
- Romaine lettuce, 5 c.
- Divide among salad bowls and serve.

Nutrition: Calories

30) Roasted vegetables

Preparation time: Cooking time: Servings: 4

Ingredients:
- Halls
- Allium (garlic) powder, 1 tablespoon
- Coconut oil, 1 tablespoon
- Pepper - crushed, yellow bell, one
- Pepper - crushed, red bell, one

Ingredients:
- Chopped carrot, one
- Cut asparagus, .5 bunch
- Cherry tomatoes, 1 pint
- Halved mushrooms, .5 c.

Directions:
- You need to heat the oven to 425.
- Place the carrot, peppers, tomatoes, mushrooms and asparagus in a large bowl.
- In another bowl, place the garlic powder, sodium chloride and coconut milk. Mix well.
- Pass over the vegetables and stir to coat.
- Pour vegetables onto a cooking wrap and place on the stove for 15 minutes until vegetables are tender.
- Divide among four plates and enjoy.

Nutrition: Calories

31) Pad Thai Salad

Preparation time: Cooking time: Servings: 2

Ingredients:
- Salt, .5 tsp
- Stevia, 1 packet
- Tamarind paste, 1 teaspoon
- Chopped garlic, 1 clove
- Juice of a lime
- Chopped almonds, 2 tablespoons

Ingredients:
- Chopped shallot, 1
- Peeled zucchini, 1
- Thinly sliced carrot, 2
- Bean sprouts, 1 c.
- Iceberg lettuce, 4 c.

Directions:
- Place the almonds, bean sprouts, zucchini, carrots and lettuce in a large bowl.
- Place the salt, stevia, lime juice, tamarind paste and garlic in a small food processor. Process until well blended.
- Pour the dressing over the vegetables and toss to coat.
- Divide evenly among serving bowls.

Nutrition: Calories

32) Cucumber salad

Preparation time: Cooking time: Servings: 4

Ingredients:
- Pepper
- Halls
- Sesame seed oil, 3 tablespoons

Ingredients:
- Chopped garlic, 4 cloves
- Cucumber, 1 lb.

Directions:
- Place the pepper, salt, sesame seed oil and garlic in a bowl. Whisk well to combine. Wash cucumbers and trim ends.
- Cut them in half lengthwise and then slice them into crescents.
- Add the dressing mixture to the cucumbers and toss well to coat.
- Place in the refrigerator for ten minutes. Enjoy.

Nutrition: Calories

33) Pasta salad with red lentils

Preparation time: Cooking time: Servings: 4

Ingredients:
- For the dressing and pasta -
- Pepper, .25 tsp
- Sea salt, .25 tsp
- Dried oregano, 1 teaspoon
- Lemon juice, one tablespoon
- Apple vinegar, two tablespoons
- Avocado - oil, .25 c.
- Red lentil pasta, 2 c.

Directions:
- Cook pasta according to package directions.
- While the pasta is cooking, whisk together the pepper, salt, oregano, lemon juice, vinegar and avocado oil until well combined. Adjust the seasoning as needed.

Nutrition: Calories

Ingredients:
- Vegetables -
- Crushed garlic, 2 cloves
- Sliced summer squash, .5
- Sliced zucchini, .5
- Diced red onion, .33 c.
- Chopped bell pepper - orange, bell, 1 c.
- Chopped asparagus stalks, 6
- Avocado oil, 1 tablespoon
- For the vegetables, heat the oil in a large skillet and cook the garlic, squash, zucchini, onion, bell bell pepper and asparagus. Cook for two to three minutes, or until soft.
- Add pasta, vegetables and dressing to a bowl and toss. Divide among four plates and enjoy.

34) Salad with peach sauce

Preparation time: Cooking time: Servings: 2

Ingredients:
- Seasoning -
- Pinch of sea salt
- Lemon juice, 1 teaspoon
- Water, .25 c
- Brown rice syrup, 3 to 4 tablespoons
- Tahini, 4 tablespoons
- Sauce -
- Diced Jalapeno, .5

Directions:
- For the dressing, whisk together the salt, lemon juice, water, brown rice syrup and tahini until combined. Adjust seasonings as needed.

Nutrition: Calories

Ingredients:
- Chopped purple onion, one tablespoon
- Diced coriander, one tablespoon
- Chopped bell pepper - red, bell, .25 c.
- Peach cut into cubes and pitted
- Assembly -
- Mixed green salad - 3 c

- Mix all dressing ingredients in another container.
- To make the salad, place the green salad on two plates and cover with the dressing. Drizzle with the dressing and enjoy.

35) Pineapple salad

Preparation time: Cooking time: Servings: 1

Ingredients:
- Seasoning -
- Chopped cilantro, .5 c.
- Chopped shallots, .5 c.
- Lime juice, 2 tablespoons
- Water, .25 c.
- Avocado oil, .25 c.
- Sea salt, 0.5 teaspoons

Directions:
- Place each seasoning content in your blender and blend until well combined. Adjust seasonings as needed.

Nutrition: Calories

Ingredients:
- Garlic, 2 cloves
- Assembly -
- Dulce flakes
- Chopped purple cabbage, 1 c.
- Cubed pineapple, .5 c.
- Mixed salad, 2 c.

- To make the salad, place the green salad in a bowl and add the dulse flakes, purple cabbage and pineapple. Pour in the dressing and toss to combine. Enjoy.

36) *Sweet potato salad with Jalapeno sauce*

Preparation time: **Cooking time:** **Servings: 2**

Ingredients:
- ✓ Sweet potatoes -
- ✓ Sea salt, .25 tsp
- ✓ Paprika, 1 teaspoon
- ✓ Crushed garlic, 2 cloves
- ✓ Avocado oil, 2 tablespoons
- ✓ Sweet potatoes peeled and diced, 3
- ✓ Seasoning -
- ✓ Water, 1 c.

Directions:
- ❖ Start by setting your kitchen appliance to three hundred and fifty degrees. Place some parchment on a sheet of kitchen paper.
- ❖ Dice the sweet potatoes with the salt, paprika, garlic and avocado oil. Make sure the potatoes are well coated.

Ingredients:
- ✓ Sea salt, 0.5 teaspoons
- ✓ Lime juice, 2 tablespoons
- ✓ Jalapeno
- ✓ Cilantro leaves, .25 c.
- ✓ Raw cashews, 1 c.
- ✓ Assembly -
- ✓ Mixed salad, 2 c.

- ❖ Spread the sweet potatoes on the baking sheet and bake for 25 minutes, or until soft.
- ❖ While the potatoes are cooking, add the salt, lime juice, jalapeno, cilantro, cashews and water to a high-speed blender and blend until smooth.
- ❖ To make the salad, divide the green salad into two plates and top with the cooked sweet potatoes. Add the dressing and toss to combine.

Nutrition: Calories

37) *Asparagus salad with lemon sauce*

Preparation time: **Cooking time:** **Portions:**

Ingredients:
- ✓ Salad -
- ✓ Pepper, .25 tsp
- ✓ Sea salt, 0.5 teaspoons
- ✓ Crushed garlic, 3 cloves
- ✓ Diced onion, .5 c.
- ✓ Diced asparagus stems, 24
- ✓ Avocado oil, 1 teaspoon

Directions:
- ❖ For the asparagus, heat the oil in a massive skillet and put in the pepper, salt, garlic, onion bulb, then the asparagus. Prepare for five to seven minutes, or until the onion has become soft.
- ❖ To make the dressing, add half of the cooked asparagus mixture to a blender along with the pepper, salt, lemon juice, water and cashews.

Nutrition: Calories

Ingredients:
- ✓ Seasoning -
- ✓ Pepper
- ✓ Sea salt, .25 tsp
- ✓ Lemon juice, 2 tablespoons
- ✓ Water, .5 c.
- ✓ Raw cashews, .5 c.
- ✓ Assembly -
- ✓ Mixed salad, 2 c.

- ❖ Blend until smooth and creamy.
- ❖ To make the salad, divide the vegetable mixture between two plates and top with the rest of the cooked asparagus. Top with the dressing and enjoy.

38) Vegetarian lettuce rolls

Preparation time: 20 minutes **Cooking time**: 10 minutes **Servings**: 4

Ingredients:
- ✓ For filling:
- ✓ 1 teaspoon of olive oil
- ✓ 2 cups fresh shiitake mushrooms, chopped
- ✓ 2 teaspoons of tamari, divided
- ✓ 1 cup of cooked quinoa
- ✓ 1 teaspoon fresh lime juice
- ✓ 1 teaspoon organic apple cider vinegar
- ✓ ¼ cup shallots, chopped
- ✓ Sea salt and freshly ground black pepper, to taste
- ✓ For the creamy sauce:
- ✓ 5 ounces of silken tofu, pressed, drained and chopped
- ✓ 1 small clove of garlic, minced

Ingredients:
- ✓ ¼ cup plain almond butter
- ✓ 1 teaspoon fresh lime juice
- ✓ Sea salt and freshly ground black pepper, to taste
- ✓ For wrappers:
- ✓ 8 medium lettuce leaves
- ✓ ¼ cup cucumber, peeled and julienned
- ✓ ¼ cup of carrot, peeled and julienned
- ✓ ¼ cup of cabbage, shredded

Directions:
- ❖ For the filling, in a skillet, heat oil over medium heat and cook mushrooms and 1 teaspoon tamari for about 5-8 minutes, stirring often.
- ❖ Stir in the quinoa, lime juice, vinegar and remaining tamari and cook for about 1 minute, stirring constantly.
- ❖ Add the shallot, salt and black pepper and immediately remove from heat.
- ❖ Set aside to cool.
- ❖ Meanwhile, for the sauce: in a food processor, add all ingredients and pulse until smooth.
- ❖ Arrange the lettuce leaves on serving plates.
- ❖ Place quinoa filling evenly on each leaf and top with cucumbers, carrots and cabbage.
- ❖ Serve alongside the creamy sauce.

Nutrition: Calories

39) Oatmeal, tofu and spinach burger

Preparation time: 15 minutes **Cooking time**: 16 minutes **Servings**: 4

Ingredients:
- ✓ 1 pound firm tofu, drained, pressed and crumbled
- ✓ ¾ cup rolled oats
- ✓ ¼ cup of flaxseed
- ✓ 2 cups frozen cabbage, thawed, squeezed and shredded
- ✓ 1 medium onion, finely chopped
- ✓ 4 garlic cloves, minced

Ingredients:
- ✓ 1 teaspoon of ground cumin
- ✓ 1 teaspoon of red pepper flakes, crushed
- ✓ Sea salt and freshly ground black pepper, to taste
- ✓ 2 tablespoons of olive oil
- ✓ 6 cups of fresh salad

Directions:
- ❖ In a large bowl, add all ingredients except oil and green salads and mix until well combined.
- ❖ Set aside for about 10 minutes.
- ❖ Cut out desired size patties from the dough.
- ❖ In a nonstick skillet, heat oil over medium heat and cook patties for 6-8 minutes per side.
- ❖ Serve these patties alongside the green salad.

Nutrition: Calories

40) Hamburger with beans, nuts and vegetables

Preparation time: 20 minutes **Cooking time**: 25 minutes **Servings**: 4

Ingredients:
- ✓ ½ cup of walnuts
- ✓ 1 carrot, peeled and chopped
- ✓ 1 celery stalk, chopped
- ✓ 4 shallots, chopped
- ✓ 5 cloves of garlic, minced
- ✓ 2¼ cups canned black beans, rinsed and drained

Ingredients:
- ✓ 2½ cups sweet potato, peeled and grated
- ✓ ½ teaspoon of red pepper flakes, crushed
- ✓ ¼ teaspoon cayenne pepper
- ✓ Sea salt and freshly ground black pepper, to taste
- ✓ 12 cups of fresh vegetables

Directions:
- ❖ Preheat oven to 400 degrees F. Line a baking sheet with baking paper.
- ❖ In a food processor, add the walnuts and pulse until finely ground.
- ❖ Add the carrot, celery, shallot and garlic and chop finely.
- ❖ Transfer the vegetable mixture to a large bowl.
- ❖ In the same food processor, add the beans and pulse until chopped.
- ❖ Add 1 1/2 cups sweet potatoes and pulse until a chunky mixture forms.
- ❖ Transfer the bean mixture to the bowl with the vegetable mixture.
- ❖ Stir in the remaining sweet potato, spices, salt and black pepper and mix until well combined.
- ❖ Make 8 equal-sized patties with the bean mixture.
- ❖ Arrange the meatballs on the prepared baking sheet in a single layer.
- ❖ Bake for about 25 minutes.
- ❖ Divide vegetables among serving plates and top each with 2 meatballs.
- ❖ Serve immediately.

Nutrition: Calories

Chapter 4 - Dinner Recipes

41) Potato and broccoli soup

Preparation time: 10 minutes **Cooking time:** 25 minutes **Servings:** 2 to 1

Ingredients:
- ✓ 1 tablespoon avocado oil
- ✓ ½ cup diced onion
- ✓ 2 garlic cloves, crushed
- ✓ 3 cups of vegetable broth
- ✓ 1 (13.5-ounce / 383-g) can of whole coconut milk

Directions:
- ❖ In a large skillet over medium-high heat, heat the avocado oil. Add the onion and garlic and sauté for 2 to 3 minutes, or until the onions are soft.
- ❖ Add the vegetable broth, coconut milk, potatoes, broccoli, salt and pepper, and continue to cook for 18-20 minutes, or until the potatoes are soft. Remove from heat and cool.

Nutrition: Calories

Ingredients:
- ✓ 2 cups of potatoes peeled and cut into cubes
- ✓ 3 cups chopped broccoli florets
- ✓ 1 teaspoon of sea salt
- ✓ 1½ teaspoons of freshly ground black pepper

- ❖ In a blender, blend the cooled soup until smooth.
- ❖ Adjust seasonings as needed. Pour into 2 large or 4 small bowls and enjoy.

42) Lush bell pepper soup

Preparation time: 5 minutes **Cooking time:** 10 minutes **Servings:** from 2 to 4

Ingredients:
- ✓ 1 teaspoon of avocado oil
- ✓ ¼ cup diced onions
- ✓ 2 garlic cloves, crushed
- ✓ 2 cups of diced red peppers
- ✓ 2 cups of vegetable broth

Directions:
- ❖ In a skillet over medium-high heat, add avocado oil, onions, garlic, and red peppers, and sauté for 2 to 3 minutes, or until onions are soft; let cool.
- ❖ In a blender, blend together the soffritto, vegetable broth, jalapeño, and salt until well combined and completely liquid; adjust seasonings according to your preference.

Nutrition: Calories

Ingredients:
- ✓ ½ to 1 jalapeño, seeded and diced
- ✓ 1 teaspoon of sea salt
- ✓ ½ cup diced red peppers
- ✓ ½ cup of diced yellow peppers

- ❖ Transfer the soup to a medium bowl and toss with the diced red and yellow peppers.
- ❖ Cover and refrigerate for 20-30 minutes to chill or chill overnight.
- ❖ Pour into 2 large or 4 small bowls and enjoy.

43) Cabbage and yellow onion soup

Preparation time: 10 minutes **Cooking time:** 20 minutes **Servings:** from 2 to 4

Ingredients:
- ✓ 1 tablespoon avocado oil
- ✓ 2 cups thinly sliced yellow onions (3 medium)
- ✓ 1 teaspoon of unrefined whole cane sugar, such as Sucanat
- ✓ 1 cup of vegetable broth
- ✓ 2 cups of water

Directions:
- ❖ In a medium saucepan over medium-high heat, heat the avocado oil. Add the onions and sauté for 3-5 minutes, or until the onions begin to get soft.
- ❖ Add the sugar and continue to sauté, stirring constantly, for 8-10 minutes, or until the onions are slightly caramelized.

Nutrition: Calories

Ingredients:
- ✓ 2 tablespoons of coconut amino acids
- ✓ 2 garlic cloves, crushed
- ✓ ½ teaspoon of dried thyme
- ✓ ½ teaspoon of sea salt
- ✓ 3 cabbage stalks, shredded and cut into ribbons (about 2 cups)

- ❖ Add the vegetable broth, water, coconut amino acid, garlic, thyme, and salt. Reduce heat to medium-low and simmer for 5-7 minutes. Adjust seasonings as needed.
- ❖ Add the cabbage and leave on the heat just long enough to wilt it.
- ❖ Remove from heat, pour into 2 large or 4 small bowls and serve.

44) Wild rice, mushroom and leek soup

Preparation time: 10 minutes **Cooking time**: 55 minutes **Servings**: 1 to 2

Ingredients:
- ⅓ cup of wild rice
- 1 cup sliced cremini mushrooms
- ½ cup sliced leeks, white part only
- 3 cups of water

Directions:
- Prepare wild rice according to package instructions.
- In a medium saucepan over high heat, bring sliced mushrooms, leeks and water to a boil. Boil for 8-10 minutes, or until mushrooms are soft.

Nutrition: Calories

Ingredients:
- 2 tablespoons of organic white miso
- ¼ to ½ teaspoon freshly ground black pepper
- Sliced shallots, for garnish

- Add the cooked wild rice, miso and black pepper. Using the back side of a spoon, mash the miso on the side of the pot to break it up, then stir it in.
- Remove from heat. Pour into 1 large or 2 small bowls, garnish with chopped scallions and enjoy.

45) Pear and ginger soup

Preparation time: 10 minutes **Cooking time**: 15 minutes **Servings**: 1 to 2

Ingredients:
- 2 teaspoons of avocado oil
- ½ cup diced onions
- 2 garlic cloves, crushed
- 1 cup of vegetable broth
- 2 cups of water
- ¼ cup coconut milk (canned)

Directions:
- In a large skillet over medium-high heat, heat the avocado oil. Add the onion and garlic and sauté for 2 to 3 minutes, or until the onions are soft.
- Add the vegetable broth, water, coconut milk, pears, ginger and salt, and cook over medium-high heat for 8-10 minutes, or until the pears are soft. Remove from heat and cool.

Nutrition: Calories

Ingredients:
- 2 pears peeled and cut into cubes
- 1 inch fresh ginger root, chopped
- ¼ teaspoon of sea salt
- Sliced radishes, for garnish (optional)
- Chopped shallots, for garnish (optional)

- Transfer the soup to a blender and blend until well combined. Adjust seasonings as needed.
- Pour immediately into 1 large bowl or 2 small bowls, garnish with the radishes and scallions (if using), and enjoy, or return the soup to the stove to warm slightly over low heat before serving.

46) Asparagus and artichoke soup

Preparation time: 5 minutes **Cooking time**: 20 minutes **Servings**: 4 cups

Ingredients:
- ½ cup diced onion
- 1 tablespoon avocado oil
- 2 garlic cloves, crushed
- 1 cup of diced potatoes
- 8 asparagus stalks, cut into small pieces

Directions:
- In a medium skillet, sauté onion, avocado oil and garlic over medium-high heat for 2 to 3 minutes, or until onion is soft.
- Transfer the sauté to a medium-sized saucepan and add the potatoes, asparagus, vegetable broth, salt and pepper; cook over medium-high heat for 18 to 20 minutes, or until the potatoes are soft. Add more vegetable broth, if necessary, to keep the liquid level between ½ and 1 inch above the contents of the saucepan. Remove from heat and allow to cool.

Nutrition: Calories

Ingredients:
- 2 cups of vegetable broth
- ½ to ¾ teaspoon sea salt
- ½ teaspoon of ground black pepper
- 2 cups of almond milk
- 1 can of artichoke hearts, cut in half and with stem

- In a blender, blend the cooled soup mixture, almond milk and artichokes until everything is well combined and the soup is smooth. Adjust the seasonings to your liking and add more almond milk or vegetable broth to thin it out, if you prefer.
- Return the soup to the casserole dish and heat slightly over low heat before serving.

47) Carrot and celery soup

Preparation time: 15 minutes **Cooking time**: 1 hour and 10 minutes **Servings**: 4 people

Ingredients:
- Kitchen spray
- 1 large onion, coarsely chopped
- 2 large carrots, peeled and roughly chopped
- 2 large celery stalks (with leaves), coarsely chopped
- 1 parsnip, peeled and coarsely chopped

Directions:
- Spray the bottom of a large pot with cooking spray. Place the pot over medium-low heat, add the onion and sauté for about 5 minutes, stirring constantly.
- Add the carrots, celery, parsnips, garlic and leek to the pot. Sauté for an additional 3 minutes.

Ingredients:
- 5 cloves of garlic, crushed
- 1 leek, well cleaned and coarsely chopped
- 9 cups of water
- 2 bay leaves
- 2 teaspoons of sea salt
- Add the water, bay leaf and salt. Simmer for 1 hour.
- Remove from heat and cool slightly. Drain the vegetables, leaving only the broth.
- To serve, add back some of the vegetables if you like and heat the soup to your desired temperature.

Nutrition: Calories

48) Creamy clam chowder with mushrooms

Preparation time: 15 minutes **Cooking time**: 30 minutes **Servings**: 4

Ingredients:
- For the mushroom clams:
- ½ cup coarsely chopped shiitake mushrooms
- 1 teaspoon of coconut oil
- ¼ cup of water
- ½ teaspoon celery seeds
- For the soup base:
- ½ medium onion, chopped
- 3 medium carrots, peeled and chopped
- 2 stalks of celery, finely chopped

Directions:
- To make clams with mushrooms
- In a large pot over medium-high heat, add mushrooms and coconut oil. Sauté for 3 minutes. Add the water and celery seeds, stirring until the water is absorbed.
- Remove from heat and transfer mushrooms to a plate.
- To make the soup base
- In the same pot, over medium heat, sauté the onion, carrots, celery and thyme for about 5 minutes, or until the onion is softened. Add a little broth, if needed.

Ingredients:
- 1 teaspoon of dried thyme
- 3 cups of vegetable broth
- 1 sheet of nori, finely crumbled
- For the cream base:
- 1 cup lightly steamed cauliflower
- ¾ cup unsweetened almond milk
- ¼ teaspoon of sea salt

- Then, add the remaining broth and nori and bring to a boil.
- To make the cream base
- In a blender or food processor, add the cauliflower, almond milk and salt. Blend to combine. If the mixture is too thick, add a little soup base to thin it out. Blend until the mixture is smooth.
- To assemble the fish soup
- Add the mushroom mix and cream base to the soup base. Stir well to combine.
- Reheat for 5 minutes, or until hot, and serve.

Nutrition: Calories

49) Soup of bok choy, broccolini and brown rice

Preparation time: 5 minutes **Cooking time**: 10 minutes **Servings**: 2

Ingredients:
- 3 cups of vegetable broth
- 1 cup of chopped bok choy

Ingredients:
- 1 bunch of broccolini, coarsely chopped
- ½ cup cooked brown rice

Directions:
- In a medium saucepan over medium heat, place the broth, bok choy, broccolini and brown rice. Bring to a boil and cook for 10 minutes, or until vegetables are cooked through and tender. Serve.

Nutrition: Calories

50) Apple and sweet pumpkin soup

Preparation time: 5 minutes **Cooking time**: 25 minutes **Servings**: 2 people

Ingredients:
- 1 medium apple, core and slices
- ½ cup chopped fennel
- 1½ cups of water, divided
- 1 cup unsweetened canned pumpkin puree
- ¾ cup low-sodium vegetable broth
- 4 small dates, pitted
- 2 teaspoons of fresh grated ginger or 2 cubes of frozen ginger

Directions:
- In a saucepan, combine the apples, fennel and ½ cup water. Cover and simmer for about 25 minutes, until the apples and fennel are softened.
- In a food processor, combine the apple and fennel mixture, pumpkin, remaining 1 cup water, broth, dates, ginger, cinnamon, curry powder, thyme, salt and cumin. Process until reduced to a puree.

Nutrition: Calories

Ingredients:
- ¼ teaspoon ground cinnamon
- ¼ teaspoon of curry powder
- ⅛ teaspoon of dried thyme
- ¼ teaspoon sea salt
- ⅛ teaspoon of ground cumin
- 4 teaspoons of raisins, for garnish
- 2 teaspoons fennel seeds, toasted, for garnish

- Pour soup into two bowls and top each with 2 teaspoons raisins and 1 teaspoon toasted fennel seeds.
- Serve immediately or let cool and serve at room temperature.

51) Tomato and carrot soup with lemon

Preparation time: 5 minutes **Cooking time**: 35 minutes **Servings**: 2

Ingredients:
- 1(15-ounce / 425-g) can no sodium added diced tomatoes, drained
- ¾ cup chopped carrots
- 1 tablespoon avocado oil
- ¼ teaspoon of sea salt

Directions:
- Preheat the oven to 400°F (205°C).
- In a glass baking dish, combine the tomatoes, carrots, oil and salt and mix well.

Nutrition: Calories

Ingredients:
- 1 cup of water
- ½ cup low-sodium vegetable broth
- 2 tablespoons fresh coriander chopped
- 1 tablespoon freshly squeezed lemon juice

- Cook tomato and carrot mixture for 35 minutes, or until caramelized, then carefully transfer to a food processor.
- Add the water and broth and blend until smooth.
- Garnish with the cilantro and add lemon juice to taste.

52) Zucchini and avocado soup with basil

Preparation time: 5 minutes **Cooking time**: 0 minutes **Servings**: 2 people

Ingredients:
- 2 large zucchini, chopped
- 1 medium avocado
- 1 medium bell pepper
- ½ cup low-sodium vegetable broth
- ½ cup of water
- ¼ cup chopped fennel

Directions:
- In a high-speed blender or food processor, combine the zucchini, avocado, bell bell pepper, broth, water, fennel, basil, rosemary, garlic and salt and blend until pureed.

Nutrition: Calories

Ingredients:
- 6 fresh basil leaves, plus 2 small leaves for garnish
- 2 teaspoons fresh rosemary chopped
- 1 garlic clove, peeled, or 1 frozen garlic cube
- ⅛ teaspoon sea salt
- 1½ teaspoons hulled pumpkin seeds, toasted, for garnish

- Pour the soup into the bowls. Garnish each with a small basil leaf and the pumpkin seeds and serve.

53) Zucchini, spinach and quinoa soup

Preparation time: 5 minutes   **Cooking time**: 25 minutes   **Servings**: 4 people

Ingredients:
- 2 tablespoons of avocado oil
- ¼ teaspoon of dried oregano
- ¼ teaspoon of dried thyme
- ⅛ teaspoon sea salt
- 1 large onion, chopped
- 2 large zucchini, peeled and cut into pieces

Directions:
- In a soup pot, heat the oil over medium heat for 1 minute, then add the oregano, thyme and salt and cook for 30 seconds.
- Add onion, cover and cook for 7-8 minutes, stirring regularly, until softened.
- Add the zucchini. Cook for an additional 12 minutes, or until zucchini is soft.

Nutrition: Calories

Ingredients:
- 1 cup low-sodium vegetable broth
- 1 cup of water
- 1 cup baby spinach
- 6 large fresh basil leaves
- ⅓ cup of cooked quinoa (optional)
- Juice of 1 lemon

- Add the broth and water and cook for another 3 minutes, until heated through.
- Add the spinach and basil and cook until just wilted.
- Transfer the mixture to a food processor and process until pureed.
- Add quinoa (if using). Season with lemon juice and serve.

54) Easy Cilantro Lime Quinoa.

Preparation time: 5 minutes   **Cooking time**: 15 minutes   **Servings**: 6

Ingredients:
- 1 cup quinoa, rinsed and draned.
- ½ cup fresh cilantro, chopped
- 1 lime zest, grated

Directions:
- Add quinoa and water to the instant pot and stir well.
- Seal with a lid and select manual mode and set the timer for 5 minutes.

Nutrition: Calories

Ingredients:
- 2 tbsp. fresh lime juice
- 1 ¼ cup of distilled water feed Sea sa sa

- Once finished, allow pressure naturally release that open thed.
- Stir in water, let stand and let rest.
- Season with salt and serve.

55) Spinach Quinoa

Preparation time: 10 minutes   **Cooking time**: 25 minutes   **Servings**: 4

Ingredients:
- 1 cup quinoa
- 2 cups fresh spinach, chopped
- 1 ½ cups filtered alkaline water
- 1 sweet potato, peeled and cut into pieces
- 1 tsp. coriander powder
- 1 teaspoon of turmandine
- 1 teaspoon of cumin seds

Directions:
- Add oil il instant pot and set the sauté mode.
- Add onion in olive oil and saute for 2 minutes otil onion is softened.
- Add garlic, ginger, spices and quinoa and coook for 3-4 minutes.
- Add spinach, sweet potatoes, and water and stir well.

Nutrition: Calories

Ingredients:
- 1 tsp. fresh ginger, chopped
- 2 garlic cloves, chopped
- 1 onion cut in half
- 2 tbsp olive oil
- 1 fresh lime juice
- Pepper Salt

- Cook on high pressure for 2 minutes.
- When it's finished, release the pressure naturally and then open the container. Add the lime juice and mix well.
- Serve and enjoy.

56) Healthy broccoli soup Asparagus

Preparation time: 15 minutes. **Cooking time:** 28 minutes. **Servings: 6**

Ingredients:
- 2 cups broccoli florets, chopped
- 15 asparagus spears, es cut and chopped
- 1 tsp. dried oregano
- 1 tbsp. fresh thyme leaves
- ½ cup unsweetened almond milk

Directions:
- Add the oil to the bowl and stir the bowl.
- Add onion to olive oil and sauté until onion is softened.
- Add the garlic and let stand for 30 minutes.
- Add all the vegetables and salt and dry well.

Nutrition: Calories

Ingredients:
- 3 ½ cups filtered alkaline water
- 2 cups cauliflower florets, chopped
- 2 tsp. garlic, chopped 1 cup onion, chopped
- 2 tbsp. olive oil
- Salt Pepper
- Seal pot with lid and coook on manual mode for 3 minutes.
- Once finished, you can rinse to minimize pressure and then close the container.
- Puree the soup with an immersion blender until smooth. Add the almond milk, herbs, pepper and salt.
- Serve and enjoy.

57) Creamy Asparagus Soup

Preparation time: 10 minutes **Cooking time:** 40 minutes **Servings: 6**

Ingredients:
- 2 lbs. fresh asparagus cut off woody stems
- ¼ tablespoon of lemon zest
- 2 tbsp. lime juice
- 14 oz. coconut milk
- 1 tsp. tied thyme.
- ½ tsp. oregano
- ½ tsp. sage

Directions:
- Preheat the oven to 400°F/ 200°C.
- The paper tray with the scraps and leftovers.
- Arrange the asparagus spears on a baking sheet. Add 2 tablespoons of walnut oil and add salt, seasonings, garlic and sugar.
- Kiss it with a dose of 20-25 mnutes.
- Add the remaining oil in the instant pot and set the pot on sauté mode.
- Add the garlic and milk to the pot and saute for 2-3 minutes.

Nutrition: Calories

Ingredients:
- 1 ½ cups alkaline water filtered.
- 1 Head of a hunting dog coming out of the floor.
- 1 tablespoon. garlic, minced
- 1 leek, sliced
- 3 tbsp. coconut oil
- Pinch of Himalayan salt.
- Add the cauliflower florets and water to the bowl and mix well.
- Insert pot with a rod and select steam and let stand for 4 minutes.
- When you finished, release the pressure using the quick-release method.
- Add roasted asparagus, lime zest, lime juice, and coco milk and stir well.
- Puree the soup with an immersion blender until pureed.
- Serve and have fun

58) Spicy Eggplant

Preparation time: 15 minutes **Cooking time:** 5 minutes **Servings: 4**

Ingredients:
- 1 eggplant, cut into 1inch cubes
- ½ cup filtered alkaline water
- 1 life, in book form.
- ½ tsp. Italian seasoning
- 1 tsp. paprika

Directions:
- Add the extract and salt to the instant flour.
- Cook on manual high pressure for 5 minutes.
- When done, rinse with peanut butter and then milk. Wet eggplant well.

Nutrition: Calories

Ingredients:
- ½ tsp. red pepper
- 1 tsp. garlic powder
- 2 tbsp. olive oil extra virgin
- ¼ teaspoon of sea salt

- Add oil to the Instant Pot and set pot on sauté mode.
- Return the ingredient to the pot with the food processor, garlic, paprika, red, garlic and salt and stir until included.
- Coook on sauté mode for 5 minutes. Stir from time to time.
- Serve enjoy.

53) Zucchini, spinach and quinoa soup

Preparation time: 5 minutes   **Cooking time:** 25 minutes   **Servings:** 4 people

Ingredients:
- 2 tablespoons of avocado oil
- ¼ teaspoon of dried oregano
- ¼ teaspoon of dried thyme
- ⅛ teaspoon sea salt
- 1 large onion, chopped
- 2 large zucchini, peeled and cut into pieces

Ingredients:
- 1 cup low-sodium vegetable broth
- 1 cup of water
- 1 cup baby spinach
- 6 large fresh basil leaves
- ⅓ cup of cooked quinoa (optional)
- Juice of 1 lemon

Directions:
- In a soup pot, heat the oil over medium heat for 1 minute, then add the oregano, thyme and salt and cook for 30 seconds.
- Add onion, cover and cook for 7-8 minutes, stirring regularly, until softened.
- Add the zucchini. Cook for an additional 12 minutes, or until zucchini is soft.
- Add the broth and water and cook for another 3 minutes, until heated through.
- Add the spinach and basil and cook until just wilted.
- Transfer the mixture to a food processor and process until pureed.
- Add quinoa (if using). Season with lemon juice and serve.

Nutrition: Calories

54) Easy Cilantro Lime Quinoa.

Preparation time: 5 minutes   **Cooking time:** 15 minutes   **Servings:** 6

Ingredients:
- 1 cup quinoa, rinsed and draned.
- ½ cup fresh cilantro, chopped
- 1 lime zest, grated

Ingredients:
- 2 tbsp. fresh lime juice
- 1 ¼ cup of distilled water feed Sea sa sa

Directions:
- Add quinoa and water to the instant pot and stir well.
- Seal with a lid and select manual mode and set the timer for 5 minutes.
- Once finished, allow pressure naturally release that open thed.
- Stir in water, let stand and let rest.
- Season with salt and serve.

Nutrition: Calories

55) Spinach Quinoa

Preparation time: 10 minutes   **Cooking time:** 25 minutes   **Servings:** 4

Ingredients:
- 1 cup quinoa
- 2 cups fresh spinach, chopped
- 1 ½ cups filtered alkaline water
- 1 sweet potato, peeled and cut into pieces
- 1 tsp. coriander powder
- 1 teaspoon of turmandine
- 1 teaspoon of cumin seds

Ingredients:
- 1 tsp. fresh ginger, chopped
- 2 garlic cloves, chopped
- 1 onion cut in half
- 2 tbsp olive oil
- 1 fresh lime juice
- Pepper Salt

Directions:
- Add oil il instant pot and set the sauté mode.
- Add onion in olive oil and saute for 2 minutes otil onion is softened.
- Add garlic, ginger, spices and quinoa and coook for 3-4 minutes.
- Add spinach, sweet potatoes, and water and stir well.
- Cook on high pressure for 2 minutes.
- When it's finished, release the pressure naturally and then open the container. Add the lime juice and mix well.
- Serve and enjoy.

Nutrition: Calories

56) Healthy broccoli soup Asparagus

Preparation time: 15 minutes. **Cooking time:** 28 minutes. **Servings:** 6

Ingredients:
- 2 cups broccoli florets, chopped
- 15 asparagus spears, es cut and chopped
- 1 tsp. dried oregano
- 1 tbsp. fresh thyme leaves
- ½ cup unsweetened almond milk

Directions:
- Add the oil to the bowl and stir the bowl.
- Add onion to olive oil and sauté until onion is softened.
- Add the garlic and let stand for 30 minutes.
- Add all the vegetables and salt and dry well.

Ingredients:
- 3 ½ cups filtered alkaline water
- 2 cups cauliflower florets, chopped
- 2 tsp. garlic, chopped 1 cup onion, chopped
- 2 tbsp. olive oil
- Salt Pepper
- Seal pot with lid and coook on manual mode for 3 minutes.
- Once finished, you can rinse to minimize pressure and then close the container.
- Puree the soup with an immersion blender until smooth. Add the almond milk, herbs, pepper and salt.
- Serve and enjoy.

Nutrition: Calories

57) Creamy Asparagus Soup

Preparation time: 10 minutes **Cooking time:** 40 minutes **Servings:** 6

Ingredients:
- 2 lbs. fresh asparagus cut off woody stems
- ¼ tablespoon of lemon zest
- 2 tbsp. lime juice
- 14 oz. coconut milk
- 1 tsp. tied thyme.
- ½ tsp. oregano
- ½ tsp. sage

Directions:
- Preheat the oven to 400°F/ 200°C.
- The paper tray with the scraps and leftovers.
- Arrange the asparagus spears on a baking sheet. Add 2 tablespoons of walnut oil and add salt, seasonings, garlic and sugar.
- Kiss it with a dose of 20-25 mnutes.
- Add the remaining oil in the instant pot and set the pot on sauté mode.
- Add the garlic and milk to the pot and saute for 2-3 minutes.

Ingredients:
- 1 ½ cups alkaline water filtered.
- 1 Head of a hunting dog coming out of the floor.
- 1 tablespoon. garlic, minced
- 1 leek, sliced
- 3 tbsp. coconut oil
- Pinch of Himalayan salt.

- Add the cauliflower florets and water to the bowl and mix well.
- Insert pot with a rod and select steam and let stand for 4 minutes.
- When you finished, release the pressure using the quick-release method.
- Add roasted asparagus, lime zest, lime juice, and coco milk and stir well.
- Puree the soup with an immersion blender until pureed.
- Serve and have fun

Nutrition: Calories

58) Spicy Eggplant

Preparation time: 15 minutes **Cooking time:** 5 minutes **Servings:** 4

Ingredients:
- 1 eggplant, cut into 1inch cubes
- ½ cup filtered alkaline water
- 1 life, in book form.
- ½ tsp. Italian seasoning
- 1 tsp. paprika

Directions:
- Add the extract and salt to the instant flour.
- Cook on manual high pressure for 5 minutes.
- When done, rinse with peanut butter and then milk. Wet eggplant well.

Ingredients:
- ½ tsp. red pepper
- 1 tsp. garlic powder
- 2 tbsp. olive oil extra virgin
- ¼ teaspoon of sea salt

- Add oil to the Instant Pot and set pot on sauté mode.
- Return the ingredient to the pot with the food processor, garlic, paprika, red, garlic and salt and stir until included.
- Coook on sauté mode for 5 minutes. Stir from time to time.
- Serve enjoy.

Nutrition: Calories

59) Brussels Sprouts and carrots

Preparation time: 10 minutes   **Cooking time:** 5 minutes   **Servings:** 6

Ingredients:
- 1 1/2 pounds of Brussels sprouts, trimmed and cut alf
- 4 Carrots peel and cut slices are shaped into a knife.
- 1 tsp. olive oil
- ½ cup alkaline filtered water
- 1 tbsp. dried parsley

Ingredients:
- ¼ tsp. garlic, chopped
- ¼ tsp. pepper
- ¼ tsp. sea salt

Directions:
- Add all ingredients inside the instant pot and mix well.
- Cook the pot with the lid on and cook on high heat for 2 minutes.

- When finished, rinse with the quick release button and then the lid.
- Stir well all and serve.

Nutrition: Calories

60) Cajun Zucchini seasoned

Preparation time: 8 minutes.   **Cooking time:** 2 minutes.   **Servings:** 2

Ingredients:
- 4 zucchinis, sliced
- 1 tsp. garlic powder
- 1 tsp. paprika

Ingredients:
- 2 tbsp. Cajun seasoning
- ½ cup melted milk water
- 1 tablespoon of olive oil

Directions:
- Add all ingredients to the pot and mix well.
- Close the pot with the lid and cook on low pressure for 1 minute.
- Once finished, release the pressure using the quick-release method then opene the lid.
- Mix well and serve.
- Nutrition: Calories 130 Fat: 7.9 Carbohydrates: 14.7 g. Sugar: 7.2 g. Protein: 5.3 g. Cholesterol: 0 mg.

Chapter 5 - Snacks Recipes

61) Cracker Healthy

Preparation time: Cooking time: 30 minutes   Servings: 50 Crackers

Ingredients:
- 1/2 cup of rye flour
- 1 cup of flour Spelt
- 2 teaspoons of Sesame Seed
- 1 teaspoon of Agave Syrup

Directions:
- Preheat our oven to 350 degrees Fahrenheit.
- Add all ingredients to a glass container and mix everything together.
- Make a ball of dough. If the dough is too thick, add more flour.
- Prepare a place to spread the dough and cover it with a piece of parchment paper.
- Degrease the container well with Grape Seed Oil and put the dart in it.
- RICE the slurry with a rolling pin, adding more flour so it doesn't fall apart.

Ingredients:
- 1 teaspoon of Pure Sea Salt
- 2 tablespoons of Grape Seed Oil
- 3/4 cup of Spring Water

- When your dough is ready, take a pastry cutter and insert it into the container. If you don't have a pastry cutter, you can use a cookie cutter.
- Arrange the squares on a kitchen basket and place them in the corner of a ech square using a fork of a skewer.
- Brush the plate with a little grain oil and sprinkle with a little pure sea salt, if needed.
- Bake for 12-15 minutes or until crackers are golden brown.
- Everything that was done was done with the help of another person.
- Serve and enjoy your Healthy Crackers!

62) Tortillas

Preparation time:.   Cooking Time: 20 Minutes   Servings: 8

Ingredients:
- 2 cups of flour Spelt
- 1 teaspoon of Pure Sea Salt

Directions:
- In a food processor* blend the spelt flour with the pure salt. Blend for about 15 minutes.
- Blend, slowly add Grape seed oil until well distributed.
- Slowly add the soy water, stirring until a color forms.
- Prepare a piece of wallpaper and pour some parchment paper on it. Dust with a little flour.

Nutrition: Calories

Ingredients:
- 1/2 cup of spring Water

- Process the nut for about 1 to 2 minutes until it reaches the right consistency.
- Pour dough into 8-inch pieces.
- Roll the sandwich into a very thin shape.
- Prepare a lunch box, cook one tortilla at a time in the microwave for about 30-60 minutes.
- Serve and enjoy your Tortillas!

Helpful Hints: If you don't have a refrigerator, you can use a mixer or blender. However, you will have a better result with a food as you have nothing to do with. You can serve the Tortillas with our Sweet Butter Sauce, Avocado Sauce or Cheese. Sauce.

63) Walnut cheesecake Mango

Preparation time: Cooking time: 4 hours and 30 minutes   Servings: 8

Ingredients:
- 2 cups of Brazil Nuts
- 5 to 6 Dates
- 1 tablespoon of Sea Moss Gel (check information)
- 1/4 cup o of agave syrup
- 1/4 teaspoon salt Pure Sea
- 2 tablespoons of Lime Juice
- 1 1/2 cups of Homemade Walnut Milk *

Directions:
- Place all crust ingredients in a processor and blend for 30 seconds.
- Prepare a baking sheet with a sheet of parchment and roll out the loose dough with butter.
- Place the Mango sliced across the crust and freeze for 10 minutes.
- Place all the glass pieces in a bowl until ready.

Ingredients:
Crust:
- 1 1/2 cups of quartered Dates 1/4 cup of Agave Syrup
- 1 1/2 cups of Coconut Flakes
- 1/4 teaspoon of Pure Sea Salt
- Toppings:
- Mango of Sliced
- Sliced strawberries

- Place the filling on top of the butter, wrap it with aluminum foil or a food container and let it rest for 3 to 4 hours in the refrigerator.
- Take out dalla baking form and garnish with toppings.
- Serve and enjoy our Mango Nut Cheesecake!

64) Blackberry Jam

Preparation time: Cooking time: 4 hours and 30 minutes   Servings: 1 cup

Ingredients:
- 3/4 cup of Blackberries
- 1 tablespoon lime juice Key

Ingredients:
- 3 tablespoons of Agave Syrup
- ¼ cup of Sea Moss Gel + extra 2 tablespoons (check information)

Directions:
- ❖ Place blackberries in a medium saucepan and cook over low heat.
- ❖ Stir in blackberries until liquid is gone.
- ❖ Once you've picked the berries, use your blender to chop up the larger pieces. If you don't have a blender, put the mixture in an immersion blender, blend it well, and then return it to the oven.
- ❖ Add Sea Moss Gel, Key Lime Juice and Agave Syrup to the mixture. Cook over low heat and stir well until dry.
- ❖ Remove from heat and let sit for 10 minutes.
- ❖ Serve with pieces on flat bread.
- ❖ Enjoy your jam!

65) Blackberry Bars

Preparation time: Cooking time: 1 hour 20 Minutes Servings: 4

Ingredients:
- ✓ 3 Burro Banas or 4 Baby Banas
- ✓ 1 cup of Spelt Flour
- ✓ 2 cups of Quinoa Flakes
- ✓ 1/4 cup of Agave Syrup

Ingredients:
- ✓ 1/4 teaspoon of Pure Sea Salt
- ✓ 1/2 cup of Grape Seed Oil
- ✓ 1 cup of prepared Blackberry Jam

Directions:
- ❖ Set the oven to 350 degrees Fahrenheit.
- ❖ Mash the bananas with a fork in a large bowl.
- ❖ Combine Agave Syrup and Grape Seed Oil to the puree and mix well.
- ❖ Add the Spelt flour and Quinoa flakes. Knead the dough until it becomes sticky to your finger.
- ❖ Prepare a 9x9-inch basket with a parchment lid.
- ❖ Take 2/3 of the dough and spread it with your fingers on the baking sheet parchment pan.
- ❖ Spread Blackberry Jam over the dough.
- ❖ Crumble the rice and place it on the plate.
- ❖ Bake for 20 minutes.
- ❖ Remove from oven and let cool for 10-15 minutes.
- ❖ Cut into small pieces.
- ❖ Try and enjoy our Blackberry Bars!

66) Squash Pie.

Preparation time: Cooking time: 2 hours 30 Minutes Servings: 6-8

Ingredients:
- ✓ 2 Butternut Squashes
- ✓ 1 1/4 cups of spelt flour
- ✓ 1/4 cup of dry sugar
- ✓ 1/4 cup of Agave Syrup
- ✓ 1 teaspoon of Allspice.

Ingredients:
- ✓ 1 teaspoon of Pure Sea Salt
- ✓ 1/4 cup soy water
- ✓ 1/3 cup of fat seed oil
- ✓ 1/4 cup hemp seed milk Homemade *

Directions:
- ❖ Rinse and peel butternut pumpkins.
- ❖ Cut them in half and use a spoon to de-sed.
- ❖ Cut the meat into one piece and place in a glass container.
- ❖ Cover the squash in Spring Water and boiltare for 20-25 minutes until coooked.
- ❖ Turn off the oven and mash the cooked squash.
- ❖ Add the date sugar, agave syrup, 1/8 pure sea salt, and homemade milk and mix everything together.
- ❖ Crust:
- ❖ Preheat the oven to 350 degrees Fahrenheit.
- ❖ In a bowl, add the spelt flour, 1/2 teaspoon of Pure Sea Salt, Spring Water, and Grape Sed Oil and mix.
- ❖ Reduce the rice into a loaf of bread. Add more water or flour if needed. Let stand for 5 minutes.
- ❖ Spread out Spelt Flour on a piece of parchment paper.
- ❖ Roll out on rolling pin, adding more flour to prevent sticking.
- ❖ Place the dough in a cake pan and bake for 10 minutes.
- ❖ Remove the butter from the oven, add the filling and bake for another 40 minutes.
- ❖ Remove the cake and let it rest for 30 minutes until cool.
- ❖ Serve enjoy your Squash Pie!

Nutrition: Calories

Helpful Hints:

67) Walnut Milk homemade

Preparation time: Cooking time: minimum 8 hours Servings: 4 cups

Ingredients:
- ✓ 1 cup fresh walnuts
- ✓ 1/8 teaspoon of Pure Sea Salt

Ingredients:
- ✓ 3 cups of spring water + extra for soaking

Directions:
- ❖ Place the new Walnuts in a bag and fill it with three tablespoons of water.
- ❖ Take the Walnuts for an hour and a half.
- ❖ Drain and rinse nuts with warm water.
- ❖ Add the soaked walnuts, puree and three times the spring water to a blender.
- ❖ Mix well till smooth.
- ❖ Extend it if you need to.
- ❖ Enjoy your homemade nut milk!

Nutrition: Calories

Helpful Hints:

68) Aquafaba

Preparation time: Cooking time: 2 Hours 30 minutes Servings: 2-4 cups

Ingredients:
- 1 bag of Garbanzo beans
- 1 teaspoon of Pure Sea Salt

Directions:
- Place the chickpeas in a large pot, add the soy water and pure sea salt. Bring to a boil.
- Remove from heat and allow to soak 30 to 40 minutes.
- Strain the Garbanzo Beans and add 6 cups of water.
- Boil for 1 hour and 30 minutes on medium hat.

Nutrition: Calories

Ingredients:
- 6 cups of Spring Water + extra for soaking

- Filter the Garbanzo beans. This filtered water is Aquafaba.
- Pour the Aquafaba into a glass jar with a lid and place in the refrigerator.
- After cooling, the Aquafaba becomes thicker. If it is too thick, boil for 10-20 mnutes.

Helpful hints: Aquafaba is a good alternative for one egg: 2 tablespoons of Aquafaba = 1 egg white; 3 tablespoons of Aquafaba = 1 egg.

69) Milk Homemade Hempsed

Preparation time: Cooking time: 2 hours Servings: 2 cups

Ingredients:
- 2 tablespoons of Hemp Seeds
- 2 tablespoons of Agave Syrup

Directions:
- Place all ingredients, except fruit, in blender.
- Blend them for two minutes.
- Add fruits and resin for 30-50 minutes.

Nutrition: Calories

Helpful Hints:

Ingredients:
- 1/8 teaspoon pure salt
- 2 cups of Spring Water Fruits (optional)*.

- Store milk in the refrigerator until aged.
- Enjoy your Homemade Hempsed Milk!

70) Oil spicy infusion

Preparation time: Cooking time: 24 Hours Servings: 1 cup

Ingredients:
- ✓ **1 tablespoon of crushed Cayenne Pepper**

Directions:
- Fill a glass with a lid or bottle with grape oil.
- Add crushed Cayenne Pepper to the jar/bottle.

Ingredients:
- 3/4 cup of Grape Seed Oil

- Close and allow to cool for at least 24 hours.
- Add it to a dinner party and enjoy our Spicy Infuse oil!

71) Italian infused oil

Preparation time: Cooking time: 24 hours Servings: 1 cup

Ingredients:
- 1 teaspoon of Oregano.
- 1 teaspoon of Basil

Directions:
- Fill a glass jar with a lid or container with grape oil.
- Mix the seasonings and add them to the rice and lettuce.

Nutrition: Calories

Helpful Hints:

Ingredients:
- 1 pinch of salt Pure Sea
- 3/4 cup of Grape seed oil

- Shake and let the oil steep for at least 24 hours.
- Add it to a dish and enjoy your Infused Oil Italian!

72) Garlic Infused Oil

Preparation time: **Cooking time:** 24 hours **Servings:** 1 cup

Ingredients:
- 1/2 teaspoon of Dill
- 1/2 teaspoon of Ginger Powder
- 1 tablespoon of Onion Powder.

Directions:
- Fill a glass jar or squeeze bottle with grapeseed oil.
- Add the seasonings to the jar/bottle.

Nutrition: Calories

Helpful Hints:

Ingredients:
- 1/2 teaspoon of Pure Sea Salt
- 3/4 cup of fat seed oil
- Close and let oil infuse for at least 24 hours.
- Add it to a dish and add your "Garlic". Infused Oil!

73) Papaya Seeds Mango Dressing

Preparation time: **Cooking time:** 10 minutes **Servings:** 1/2 Cup

Ingredients:
- 1 cup of chopped Mango
- 1 teaspoon of Papaya Seeds Ground
- 1 teaspoon of Basil
- 1 teaspoon of Onion Powder

Directions:
- Prepare and place all ingredients into the mixture.
- Blend for one minute until smoth.

Nutrition: Calories

Helpful Hints:

Ingredients:
- 1 teaspoon of Agave Syrup
- 2 tablespoons of lemon juice
- 1/4 cup of grape oil
- 1/4 teaspoon salt Pure Sea
- Add it to a dish and enjoy our Papaya Seed Mango Dress5ng!

74) Blueberry Smoothie

Preparation time: 10 minutes **Cooking time:** **Servings:** 2

Ingredients:
- 2 cups of frozen blueberries
- 1 small banana

Directions:
- Place all ingredients in a high speed blender and pulse until creamy.

Nutrition: Calories

Helpful Hints:

Ingredients:
- 1½ cups unsweetened almond milk
- ¼ cup ice cubes
- Pour the smoothie into two glasses and serve immediately.

75) Raspberry and tofu smoothie

Preparation time: 10 minutes **Cooking time:** **Servings:** 2

Ingredients:
- 1½ cups of fresh raspberries
- 6 ounces of firm silken tofu, pressed and drained
- 4-5 drops of liquid stevia

Directions:
- Place all ingredients in a high speed blender and pulse until creamy.

Ingredients:
- 1 cup of coconut cream
- ¼ cup ice, crushed
- Pour the smoothie into two glasses and serve immediately.

76) Beet and Strawberry Smoothie

Preparation time: 10 minutes   **Cooking time**:   **Servings**: 2

Ingredients:
- 2 cups frozen strawberries, pitted and chopped
- ⅔ cup roasted and frozen beet, chopped
- 1 teaspoon fresh ginger, peeled and grated

Ingredients:
- 1 teaspoon fresh turmeric, peeled and grated
- ½ cup of fresh orange juice
- 1 cup unsweetened almond milk

❖ Pour the smoothie into two glasses and serve immediately.

Directions:
❖ Place all ingredients in a high speed blender and pulse until creamy.

Nutrition: Calories

Helpful Hints:

77) Kiwi Smoothie

Preparation time: 10 minutes   **Cooking time**:   **Servings**: 2

Ingredients:
- 4 kiwis
- 2 small bananas, peeled
- 1½ cups unsweetened almond milk

Ingredients:
- 1-2 drops of liquid stevia
- ¼ cup ice cubes

❖ Pour the smoothie into two glasses and serve immediately.

Directions:
❖ Place all ingredients in a high speed blender and pulse until creamy.

Nutrition: Calories

Helpful Hints:

78) Pineapple and Carrot Smoothie

Preparation time: 10 minutes   **Cooking time**:   **Servings**: 2

Ingredients:
- 1 cup frozen pineapple
- 1 large ripe banana, peeled and sliced
- ½ tablespoon fresh ginger, peeled and chopped
- ¼ teaspoon ground turmeric

Ingredients:
- 1 cup unsweetened almond milk
- ½ cup fresh carrot juice
- 1 tablespoon fresh lemon juice

❖ Pour the smoothie into two glasses and serve immediately.

Directions:
❖ Place all ingredients in a high speed blender and pulse until creamy.

Nutrition: Calories

Helpful Hints:

79) Oatmeal and orange smoothie

Preparation time: 10 minutes   **Cooking time**:   **Servings**: 4

Ingredients:
- ⅔ cup of rolled oats
- 2 oranges, peeled, seeds removed and cut into sections
- 2 large bananas, peeled and sliced

Ingredients:
- 2 cups of unsweetened almond milk
- 1 cup ice cubes, crushed

❖ Pour the smoothie into four glasses and serve immediately.

Directions:
❖ Place all ingredients in a high speed blender and pulse until creamy.

Nutrition: Calories

Helpful Hints:

80) Pumpkin Smoothie

Preparation time: 10 minutes **Cooking time**: **Servings**: 2

Ingredients:
- 1 cup homemade pumpkin puree
- 1 medium banana, peeled and sliced
- 1 tablespoon maple syrup
- 1 teaspoon ground flax seeds

Directions:
- Place all ingredients in a high speed blender and pulse until creamy.

Nutrition: Calories

Ingredients:
- ½ teaspoon ground cinnamon
- ¼ teaspoon ground ginger
- 1½ cups unsweetened almond milk
- ¼ cup ice cubes
- Pour the smoothie into two glasses and serve immediately.

Chapter 6 - Dessert Recipes

81) Red fruit and vegetable smoothie

Preparation time: 10 minutes **Cooking time**: **Servings**: 2

Ingredients:
- ½ cup fresh raspberries
- ½ cup fresh strawberries
- ½ red bell pepper, seeded and chopped
- ½ cup red cabbage, chopped

Directions:
- Place all ingredients in a high speed blender and pulse until creamy.

Nutrition: Calories

Ingredients:
- 1 small tomato
- 1 cup of water
- ½ cup of ice cubes

- Pour the smoothie into two glasses and serve immediately.

82) Kale Smoothie

Preparation time: 10 minutes **Cooking time**: **Servings**: 2

Ingredients:
- 3 fresh cabbage stalks, cut and chopped
- 1-2 celery stalks, chopped
- ½ avocado, peeled, pitted and chopped

Directions:
- Place all ingredients in a high speed blender and pulse until creamy.

Nutrition: Calories

Ingredients:
- ½ inch ginger root, chopped
- ½ inch turmeric root, chopped
- 2 cups of coconut milk

- Pour the smoothie into two glasses and serve immediately.

83) Green Tofu Smoothie

Preparation time: 10 minutes **Cooking time**: **Servings**: 2

Ingredients:
- 1½ cups cucumber, peeled and coarsely chopped
- 3 cups fresh spinach
- 2 cups of frozen broccoli
- ½ cup silken tofu, drained and pressed

Directions:
- Place all ingredients in a high speed blender and pulse until creamy.

Nutrition: Calories

Ingredients:
- 1 tablespoon fresh lime juice
- 4-5 drops of liquid stevia
- 1 cup unsweetened almond milk
- ½ cup ice, crushed
- Pour the smoothie into two glasses and serve immediately.

84) Grape and chard smoothie

Preparation time: 10 minutes **Cooking time**: **Servings**: 2

Ingredients:
- 2 cups of green grapes without seeds
- 2 cups fresh beets, cut and chopped
- 2 tablespoons of maple syrup

Directions:
- Place all ingredients in a high speed blender and pulse until creamy.

Nutrition: Calories

Ingredients:
- 1 teaspoon fresh lemon juice
- 1½ cups of water
- 4 ice cubes

- Pour the smoothie into two glasses and serve immediately.

85) Matcha Smoothie

Preparation time: 10 minutes   **Cooking time**:   **Servings**: 2

Ingredients:
- 2 tablespoons of chia seeds
- 2 teaspoons of matcha green tea powder
- ½ teaspoon fresh lemon juice
- ½ teaspoon xanthan gum

Directions:
- Place all ingredients in a high speed blender and pulse until creamy.

Nutrition: Calories

Ingredients:
- 8-10 drops of liquid stevia
- 4 tablespoons of coconut cream
- 1½ cups unsweetened almond milk
- ¼ cup ice cubes
- Pour the smoothie into two glasses and serve immediately.

86) Banana Smoothie

Preparation time: 10 minutes   **Cooking time**:   **Servings**: 2

Ingredients:
- 2 cups of cooled unsweetened almond milk
- 1 large frozen banana, peeled and sliced

Directions:
- Place all ingredients in a high speed blender and pulse until creamy.

Nutrition: Calories

Ingredients:
- 1 tablespoon almonds, chopped
- 1 teaspoon of organic vanilla extract
- Pour the smoothie into two glasses and serve immediately.

87) Strawberry Smoothie

Preparation time: 10 minutes   **Cooking time**:   **Servings**: 2

Ingredients:
- 2 cups of cooled unsweetened almond milk
- 1½ cups of frozen strawberries

Directions:
- Add all ingredients to a high speed blender and pulse until smooth.

Nutrition: Calories

Ingredients:
- 1 banana, peeled and sliced
- ¼ teaspoon of organic vanilla extract
- Pour the smoothie into two glasses and serve immediately.

88) Raspberry and tofu smoothie

Preparation time: 15 minutes   **Cooking time**:   **Servings**: 2

Ingredients:
- 1½ cups of fresh raspberries
- 6 ounces of firm silken tofu, drained
- 1/8 teaspoon of coconut extract

Directions:
- Add all ingredients to a high speed blender and pulse until smooth.

Nutrition: Calories

Ingredients:
- 1 teaspoon of stevia powder
- 1½ cups unsweetened almond milk
- ¼ cup ice cubes, crushed
- Pour the smoothie into two glasses and serve immediately.

89) Mango Smoothie

Preparation time: 10 minutes **Cooking time:** **Servings:** 2

Ingredients:
- 2 cups frozen mango, peeled, pitted and chopped
- ¼ cup almond butter
- Pinch of ground turmeric

Directions:
- Add all ingredients to a high speed blender and pulse until smooth.

Nutrition: Calories

Ingredients:
- 2 tablespoons fresh lemon juice
- 1¼ cup unsweetened almond milk
- ¼ cup ice cubes
- Pour the smoothie into two glasses and serve immediately.

90) Pineapple Smoothie

Preparation time: 10 minutes **Cooking time:** **Servings:** 2

Ingredients:
- 2 cups pineapple, chopped
- ½ teaspoon fresh ginger, peeled and chopped
- ½ teaspoon ground turmeric
- 1 teaspoon of natural immune support supplement*.

Directions:
- Add all ingredients to a high speed blender and pulse until smooth.

Nutrition: Calories

Ingredients:
- 1 teaspoon of chia seeds
- 1½ cups of cold green tea
- ½ cup ice, crushed
- Pour the smoothie into two glasses and serve immediately.

91) Cabbage and pineapple smoothie

Preparation time: 15 minutes **Cooking time:** **Servings:** 2

Ingredients:
- 1½ cups fresh cabbage, chopped and shredded
- 1 frozen banana, peeled and chopped
- ½ cup of fresh pineapple chunks

Directions:
- Add all ingredients to a high speed blender and pulse until smooth.

Nutrition: Calories

Ingredients:
- 1 cup unsweetened coconut milk
- ½ cup of fresh orange juice
- ½ cup of ice
- Pour the smoothie into two glasses and serve immediately.

92) Green Vegetable Smoothie

Preparation time: 15 minutes **Cooking time:** **Servings:** 2

Ingredients:
- 1 medium avocado, peeled, pitted and chopped
- 1 large cucumber, peeled and chopped
- 2 fresh tomatoes, chopped
- 1 small green bell pepper, seeded and chopped

Directions:
- Add all ingredients to a high speed blender and pulse until smooth.

Nutrition: Calories

Ingredients:
- 1 cup fresh spinach, torn
- 2 tablespoons fresh lime juice
- 2 tablespoons of homemade vegetable broth
- 1 cup of alkaline water
- Pour smoothie into glasses and serve immediately.

93) Avocado and spinach smoothie

Preparation time: 10 minutes **Cooking time**: **Servings**: 2

Ingredients:
- 2 cups of fresh spinach
- ½ avocado, peeled, pitted and chopped
- 4-6 drops of liquid stevia

Directions:
- Add all ingredients to a high speed blender and pulse until smooth.

Nutrition: Calories

Ingredients:
- ½ teaspoon ground cinnamon
- 1 tablespoon of hemp seeds
- 2 cups of cooled alkaline water
- Pour the smoothie into two glasses and serve immediately.

94) Cucumber Smoothie

Preparation time: 15 minutes **Cooking time**: **Servings**: 2

Ingredients:
- 1 small cucumber, peeled and chopped
- 2 cups fresh mixed greens (spinach, kale, chard), chopped and shredded
- ½ cup of lettuce, torn
- ¼ cup fresh parsley leaves
- ¼ cup fresh mint leaves

Directions:
- Add all ingredients to a high speed blender and pulse until smooth.

Nutrition: Calories

Ingredients:
- 2-3 drops of liquid stevia
- 1 teaspoon fresh lemon juice
- 1½ cups of filtered water
- ¼ cup ice cubes

- Pour the smoothie into two glasses and serve immediately.

95) Apple and Ginger Smoothie

Preparation time: 10 minutes **Cooking time**: 0 minutes **Servings**: 1

Ingredients:
- 1 apple, peeled and diced
- ¾ cup (6 ounces) of coconut yogurt

Directions:
- Add all ingredients to a blender.
- Blend well until smooth.

Nutrition: Calories

Ingredients:
- ½ teaspoon of ginger, freshly grated

- Refrigerate for 2 to 3 hours.
- Serve.

96) Green Tea Blueberry Smoothie

Preparation time: 10 minutes **Cooking time**: 5 minutes **Servings**: 1

Ingredients:
- 3 tablespoons of alkaline water
- 1 green tea bag
- 1 ½ cups fresh blueberries

Directions:
- Boil 3 tablespoons of water in a small saucepan and transfer to a cup.
- Dip the tea bag into the cup and let it sit for 4 to 5 minutes.
- Discard the tea bag and
- Transfer the green tea to a blender

Nutrition: Calories

Ingredients:
- 1 pear, peeled, stoned and diced
- ¾ cup of almond milk

- Add all other ingredients to blender.
- Blend well until smooth.
- Serve with fresh blueberries.

97) Apple and almond smoothie

Preparation time: 10 minutes Cooking time: 0 minutes Servings: 1

Ingredients:
- 1 cup of apple cider
- 1/2 cup of coconut yogurt
- 4 tablespoons almonds, crushed

Ingredients:
- 1/4 teaspoon of cinnamon
- 1/4 teaspoon nutmeg
- 1 cup of ice cubes

Directions:
- Add all ingredients to a blender.
- Blend well until smooth.
- Serve.

Nutrition: Calories

98) Cranberry Smoothie

Preparation time: 10 minutes Cooking time: 0 minutes Servings: 1

Ingredients:
- 1 cup of cranberries
- ¾ cup of almond milk
- ¼ cup raspberries

Ingredients:
- 2 teaspoons fresh ginger, finely grated
- 2 teaspoons of fresh lemon juice

Directions:
- Add all ingredients to a blender.
- Blend well until smooth.
- Serve with fresh berries on top.

Nutrition: Calories

99) Berry and Cinnamon Smoothie

Preparation time: 10 minutes Cooking time: 0 minutes Servings: 1

Ingredients:
- 1 cup of frozen strawberries
- 1 cup apple, peeled and diced
- 2 teaspoons fresh ginger
- 3 tablespoons of hemp seeds

Ingredients:
- 1 cup of water
- ½ squeezed lime
- ¼ teaspoon of cinnamon powder
- ⅛ teaspoon of vanilla extract

Directions:
- Add all ingredients to a blender.
- Blend well until smooth.
- Serve with fresh fruit

Nutrition: Calories

100) Detoxifying Berry Smoothie

Preparation time: 10 minutes Cooking time: 0 minutes Servings: 1

Ingredients:
- 3 peaches, with stone and peel
- 5 blueberries

Ingredients:
- 5 raspberries
- 1 cup of alkaline water

Directions:
- Add all ingredients to a blender.
- Blend well until smooth.
- Serve with fresh kiwi wedges.

Nutrition: Calories

Chapter 7 - Project   Chapter 7 - Dr. Lewis's Meal Plan

Day 1

1) Mile Porridge
25) Zucchini salad
47) Carrot and celery soup
61) Cracker Healthy
33) Pasta salad with red lentils

Day 2

11) Cracker Pumpkin Spice
32) Cucumber salad
41) Potato and broccoli soup
68) Aquafaba
53) Zucchini, spinach and quinoa soup

Day 3

17) Cracker Healthy
39) Oatmeal, tofu and spinach burger
58) Spicy Eggplant
67) Walnut Milk homemade
31) Pad Thai Salad

Day 4

4) Squash Hash
22) Artichoke pie
55) Spinach Quinoa   2
77) Kiwi Smoothie
45) Pear and ginger soup

Day 5

6) Veggie Medley
27) Potato and pumpkin meatballs
45) Pear and ginger soup   2
79) Oatmeal and orange smoothie
29) Southern Salad

Day 6

6) Veggie Medley
39) Oatmeal, tofu and spinach burger
60) Cajun Zucchini seasoned   2
52) Zucchini and avocado soup with basil
21) Roasted artichoke salad

Day 7

13) Wheat Crackers
26) Fried tofu
50) Apple and sweet pumpkin soup
65) Blackberry Bars
36) Sweet potato salad with Jalapeno sauce

97) Apple and almond smoothie

Preparation time: 10 minutes Cooking time: 0 minutes Servings: 1

Ingredients:
- 1 cup of apple cider
- 1/2 cup of coconut yogurt
- 4 tablespoons almonds, crushed

Directions:
- Add all ingredients to a blender.

Ingredients:
- 1/4 teaspoon of cinnamon
- 1/4 teaspoon nutmeg
- 1 cup of ice cubes
- Blend well until smooth.
- Serve.

Nutrition: Calories

98) Cranberry Smoothie

Preparation time: 10 minutes Cooking time: 0 minutes Servings: 1

Ingredients:
- 1 cup of cranberries
- ¾ cup of almond milk
- ¼ cup raspberries

Directions:
- Add all ingredients to a blender.

Ingredients:
- 2 teaspoons fresh ginger, finely grated
- 2 teaspoons of fresh lemon juice
- Blend well until smooth.
- Serve with fresh berries on top.

Nutrition: Calories

99) Berry and Cinnamon Smoothie

Preparation time: 10 minutes Cooking time: 0 minutes Servings: 1

Ingredients:
- 1 cup of frozen strawberries
- 1 cup apple, peeled and diced
- 2 teaspoons fresh ginger
- 3 tablespoons of hemp seeds

Directions:
- Add all ingredients to a blender.

Ingredients:
- 1 cup of water
- ½ squeezed lime
- ¼ teaspoon of cinnamon powder
- ⅛ teaspoon of vanilla extract
- Blend well until smooth.
- Serve with fresh fruit

Nutrition: Calories

100) Detoxifying Berry Smoothie

Preparation time: 10 minutes Cooking time: 0 minutes Servings: 1

Ingredients:
- 3 peaches, with stone and peel
- 5 blueberries

Directions:
- Add all ingredients to a blender.

Ingredients:
- 5 raspberries
- 1 cup of alkaline water
- Blend well until smooth.
- Serve with fresh kiwi wedges.

Nutrition: Calories

Chapter 7 - Project   Chapter 7 - Dr. Lewis's Meal Plan

Day 1

1) Mile Porridge
25) Zucchini salad
47) Carrot and celery soup
61) Cracker Healthy
33) Pasta salad with red lentils

Day 2

11) Cracker Pumpkin Spice
32) Cucumber salad
41) Potato and broccoli soup
68) Aquafaba
53) Zucchini, spinach and quinoa soup

Day 3

17) Cracker Healthy
39) Oatmeal, tofu and spinach burger
58) Spicy Eggplant
67) Walnut Milk homemade
31) Pad Thai Salad

Day 4

4) Squash Hash
22) Artichoke pie
55) Spinach Quinoa   2
77) Kiwi Smoothie
45) Pear and ginger soup

Day 5

6) Veggie Medley
27) Potato and pumpkin meatballs
45) Pear and ginger soup   2
79) Oatmeal and orange smoothie
29) Southern Salad

Day 6

6) Veggie Medley
39) Oatmeal, tofu and spinach burger
60) Cajun Zucchini seasoned   2
52) Zucchini and avocado soup with basil
21) Roasted artichoke salad

Day 7

13) Wheat Crackers
26) Fried tofu
50) Apple and sweet pumpkin soup
65) Blackberry Bars
36) Sweet potato salad with Jalapeno sauce

Chapter 8 - Chapter 8 - Conclusion

I hope this book can lead you to your goals, keeping your desire to keep going high, without making you lose sight of the outcome

This book series is designed to help women, men, athletes and sportsmen, people immersed in work with little free time, etc.

If you recognize yourself in one of these categories or someone you know has decided to take the same path as you,

You'll find the other books in the series in your trusted bookstore, guaranteed!

Big hugs from Dr. Grace!

CPSIA information can be obtained
at www.ICGtesting.com
Printed in the USA
BVHW050222020621
608547BV00003B/397